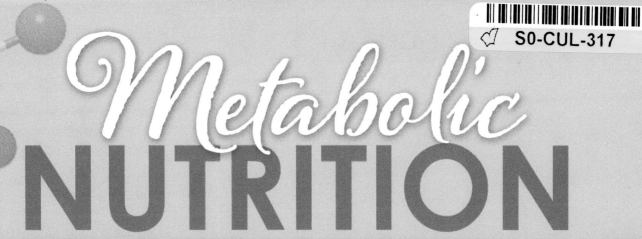

Metabolic NUTRITION

An Everyday Approach to Macronutrient Metabolism

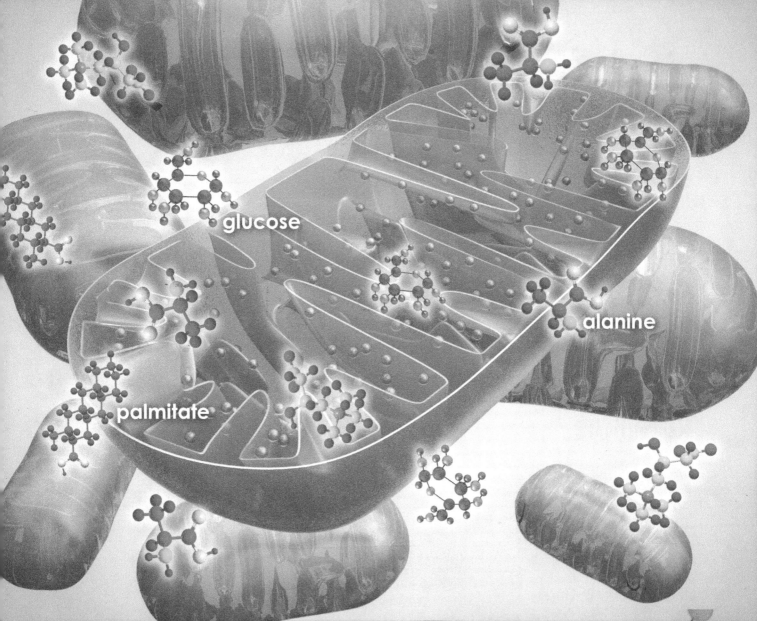

glucose

alanine

palmitate

Kendall Hunt
publishing company

Deborah Good • Matthew Hulver • Angela Anderson

Cover image © Shutterstock.com

Kendall Hunt
publishing company

www.kendallhunt.com
Send all inquiries to:
4050 Westmark Drive
Dubuque, IA 52004-1840

Copyright © 2018 by Kendall Hunt Publishing Company

ISBN: 978-1-5249-4762-0

Published in the United States of America

CONTENTS

Metabolism is complicated! A simple definition of metabolism is that it is the process of generating energy for an organism to sustain life. Metabolism consists of thousands of chemical reactions, many occurring simultaneously, for the sole purpose of ensuring an organism has ample amounts of energy to survive and thrive. Specifically, the term energy refers to a molecule termed adenosine triphosphate (ATP), which is the energy currency for all the cells in your body. In this book, you will learn more about ATP and the multiple ways that cells can produce and use it.

Our goal in writing this book is to present metabolism using a less complicated and more applicable approach. For example, we all eat meals throughout the day, have periods of 8-12 hours (perhaps even longer) when we do not eat, engage in physical activity, whether it be planned exercise or just walking around your home or at work. All of these situations affect metabolism differently. In this book, we present metabolism under these different situations. We talk about what happens from the time you take a bite of food, how your body digests the food, transports the nutrients to cells in your body, and stores it for later use. We talk about what happens after your body has processed your most recent meal, and it needs to start relying on stored energy. We discuss how your body responds to and provides the needed energy when you go from sitting to standing, resting to exercising, and how your body's metabolism changes in response to exercise training. Lastly, we talk about how your body responds when you consume more energy (food) than it needs, and we describe metabolism in context of metabolic diseases such as obesity and diabetes.

From many years of experience teaching students in the classroom, we have found it helpful to students to learn and understand metabolism when it is presented in the context of a real-life situations. Forcing the memorization of specific pathways is not conducive to retaining the information and being able to apply it to future learning opportunities and/or work-life situations. To our knowledge, this is the first textbook to present metabolism is this applicable manner. We hope you find this approach useful, interesting, and wanting to learn more about the exciting field of metabolism.

Introduction to Macronutrients

CHAPTER 1

What is Metabolism Anyway?

What is metabolism? The term "metabolism" refers to the life-sustaining processes that keep us alive. "Metabolic processes" are the enzymatic reactions that make products that living organisms need to survive. "Metabolic nutrition" is a term that characterizes the intersection between the food we eat, and the metabolic processes that turn that food intake into energy.

Everyone eats…what, why, how, and when do you eat, and how eating affects your metabolism, is the gist of this textbook. Macronutrients serve as the energy source that your body needs to produce adenosine triphosphate (ATP). If your body ceases to produce ATP, everything shuts down. To say it another way, if an organism does not eat, it won't get the nutrients it needs to be able to make ATP. While not immediate, the organism will DIE. As shown in Figure 1.1, the structure of ATP is unique, and interesting, in that the combination of phosphate groups (PO$_4$) with a nucleoside backbone means that ATP can get around the cell, shuttling from the nucleus to the cytoplasm and to cellular organelles and back again.

Take a look at a nutrition label

The FDA mandates the components of nutrition labels on foods sold in the United States. Look at a couple of these in your cupboard, and compare the protein, fat, and carbohydrate contents of foods. The label also provides information on the percent of macronutrients that the food contains, based on dietary guidelines, set by the Food and Nutrition Board.

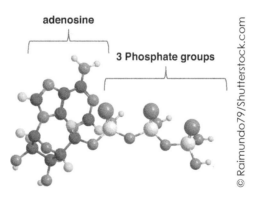

adenosine

3 Phosphate groups

© Raimundo79/Shutterstock.com

Figure 1.1: **The Structure of Adenosine Triphosphate "ATP."** ATP is composed of one adenosine, and three phosphate molecules (PO$_4$). Adenosine is a nucleoside, which is composed of the nucleotide "adenine" and one sugar "ribose". Other related molecules include adenosine diphosphate (ADP), and adenosine monophosphate (AMP), both of which are missing one additional phosphate group.

When making ATP, neither macro- nor micronutrients are sufficient alone, and as you will see, these nutrients will work together to run all of the body's systems. The pathways discussed in this textbook are activated when you eat a meal. Some are even stimulated when you don't eat, or when you exercise, or even when someone has too many nutrients available (i.e., after finishing your third plate at the local buffet restaurant, or after the Thanksgiving dinner). Conditions, such as diabetes, cancer, cardiovascular disease, inborn errors of metabolism, and others can influence how we metabolize macronutrients and influence our body's nutritional needs. In addition, environmental conditions, such as cold exposure, toxins, day or nighttime, among others can influence how our metabolic processes work. Even sitting versus standing can affect metabolic processes in your muscles and other organs. Think about that as you are reading this chapter—are you sitting down or using a standing desk? Have you recently eaten or are you hungry?

As you will see in this first chapter, food-containing (or even supplemental) macronutrients can be further divided into the organic or carbon-containing molecules: proteins, carbohydrates, and fats. These molecules will again be further divided into types of proteins, types of carbohydrates, and types of fats, the importance of which will become clear as we delve further into the material.

What is Metabolic Regulation?

Is metabolic regulation the state of "everything working properly in our bodies?", or the "ability to absorb and use nutrients?", or something else entirely? Actually, metabolic regulation is much more complex. We need to think about metabolic regulation in terms of the time period we are looking at as well as the stressors that are influencing the individual at any given time (Figure 1.2). And since metabolism can be further divided into anabolic and catabolic processes—or those processes that store (anabolic) and those that break-down (catabolic), both the forward and backwards processes need to be considered.

In regards to time period, we need to determine whether we are measuring metabolic regulation in terms of seconds, minutes, hours (short-term) or days, weeks, months, and a lifetime (long-term)?

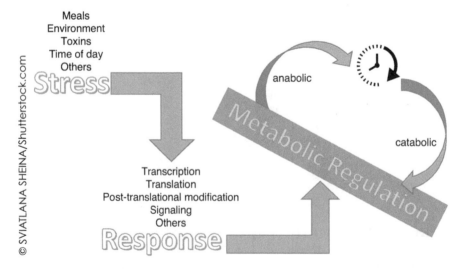

Figure 1.2: **Metabolic Regulation.** Stressors are anything that can influence metabolic regulation. These stressors instigate a response, which can change overall metabolic regulation. However, the current ongoing anabolic and catabolic processes, as well as the length of time we are measuring, can influence the magnitude of response that is measured.

The ability of our bodies, and the metabolic processes in each of our tissues to provide ATP each second, minute, hour, and day and to ensure that each organ and body system has adequate energy stores to continue to function through our lifetimes is the key to the importance of metabolic regulation.

The term metabolic regulation also implies response to a stressor. Stressors disrupt the balance, or homeostasis, and our body's attempt to restore this balance so that enzymatic processes to sustain life, continue. For example, eating a meal can be a stressor, albeit a short-term one that needs to be responded to immediately as the nutrients enter the digestive tract and are absorbed. When you stand up after sitting down for a while, your cells must have ATP to meet this demand on our muscles. This is another short-term stressor that must be responded to and balanced. On the other hand, long-term metabolic regulation refers to physiological adaptation to stressors that occur over days or even longer. For example, continuously eating an excess of 1000 more in total calories for several weeks could be a long-term stressor. Moving to a city where you might be exposed to pollutants or toxins that modulate metabolism would require long-term metabolic regulation. For both of these long-term stressors, the body and its metabolic systems will emulate changes over the long-term. These changes are different from those that would occur immediately after you eat a meal with an excess of 1000 calories, or standing up after sitting.

While we often think of "metabolism" as referring to the whole body, metabolic regulatory responses occur at the cellular level, through transcriptional, translational, and post-translational changes involving enzymes. As shown in Figure 1.3, individual cells in our body will transcribe genes into mRNA, and this mRNA will be translated into proteins (enzymes), and the proteins can be further modulated by post-translational modifications (PTM) (such as phosphorylation during signaling processes) that can increase or decrease enzymatic activity of the protein. In fact, as we will see in the later chapters of this textbook, PTMs of metabolic enzymes are the most common

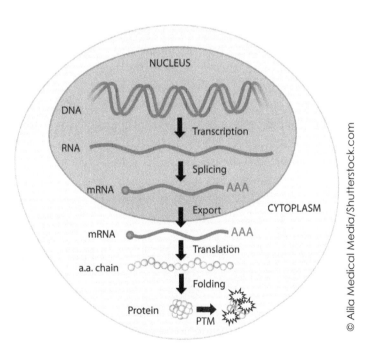

Figure 1.3: **The Central Dogma of DNA.** DNA is transcribed into mRNA, which is spliced, and then transported to the cytoplasm for protein translation. Once the new enzyme is made it can be modified by post-translational modifications (PTM). Each of these steps can be subject to metabolic regulation.

response to short-term stressors. PTMs can be transient (i.e. fall off after a certain amount of time), and usually are covalently-linked to the amino acids within proteins.

On a longer time-scale than compared to that of PTMs, transcription of genes in response to a stressor plays a major role in metabolic regulation. Transcription involves interaction of transcription factors (i.e. DNA-binding proteins) to the promoter regions of genes. Promoters of genes don't code for the protein but are usually found upstream of the start site for transcription or in other non-coding regions called enhancers. Binding of transcription factors to the promoter can either up- or down-regulate expression of that gene—resulting in either higher or lower levels of mRNA produced, and ultimately increasing or decreasing the total amount of proteins (enzymes or other proteins such as ion channels or receptors) that are made from the gene.

Making proteins from mRNA (translation) begins in the nucleus with splicing out introns from the pre-RNA, adding a 5' cap, and a poly A tail. Once in the cytoplasm, translation begins on the processed mRNA to make proteins on ribosomes. Both of these processes (splicing and translation) can be regulated. Introns, for example, can be differentially-spliced to produce different proteins from the same pre-mRNA. The mRNA itself can be degraded faster than it can be translated, or it can be stabilized by RNA-binding proteins that allow multiple proteins to be made from a single mRNA. And, the ability of ribosomes to translate mRNA into proteins can be up- or down-regulated, depending on the metabolic state of the cell and its needs.

Post-translation modifications, as mentioned above are key to both metabolic regulation, as well as to regulation of transcription, splicing, and translation of

> ## New methodologies/new insights into metabolism
>
> RNA-seq can allow researchers to investigate single-cell RNA splicing. In recent work, they found that splicing and transcription are linked and can occur simultaneously. However, and of interest to metabolic regulation, in some cases, splicing complexes can be used to slow down or even pause transcription, which could change which enzymes are produced and when. See the review article by Alpert and colleagues, 2017[1] for more information.

the genes and proteins that are needed for the metabolic response. How? PTMs affect enzymes by changing the shape of an enzyme, thereby changing its functional activity, or even its interaction with other enzymes and substrates. Allosteric regulation is further defined as the regulation of an enzyme through interaction with positive- and negative-effector molecules at positive- and negative-allosteric sites on the enzyme (Figure 1.4). Since that was a mouthful, let us look at this in more detail. The allosteric sites are *not* the substrate binding, or active site of the enzyme. However, these allosteric sites can affect whether the substrate can bind, or if the enzyme can actively process the substrate (i.e. enzymatic activity), or if the enzymes can interact with co-enzymes. The key point about allosteric regulators is that even if the proteins are already made and doing their thing, allosteric regulators can modify the enzymatic activity immediately upon sensing metabolic needs. Typically, allosteric regulators are products of an enzyme, that feed-back upon that enzyme to modulate enzyme activity. Enzyme activity can also be altered by covalent PTMs such as phosphorylation by another enzyme (a kinase in the case of phosphorylation) acting on the enzyme. It is important to note that phosphorylation sometimes increases enzymatic activity and sometimes it decreases enzymatic activity, depending on the enzyme.

There is still much to be discover and understand about metabolic regulation, especially and how the body senses and responds to changes (stressors). For example, there are many types of PTMs aside from phosphorylation (i.e, glycosylation, acetylation, sumoylation, methylation, O-glyc-N-Acylation, hydroxylation, and many, many more) that can affect metabolic regulation, but the technologies to study se many metabolic regulators are just now being developed. The ultimate role of metabolic regulation

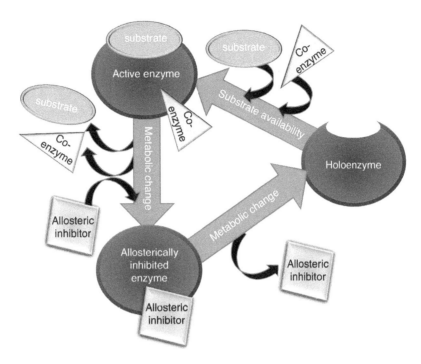

Figure 1.4: **Allosteric Regulation of an Enzyme.** In response to a metabolic change, an active enzyme can be quickly converted to an allosterically inhibited enzyme by an allosteric inhibitor. In this example, both the substrate binding area, and the ability of the co-enzyme to bind is blocked. Another metabolic change can lead to production of the holoenzyme, which is ready to be enzymatically active as soon as substrate is available.

is to meet the body's energy needs, as well as provide for storage of energy that might be needed at a later time. As we work through these metabolic processes, we'll see that the effects of stressors can be altered by the current state of the individual, in terms of its energy balance. Let's look at energy balance next.

Energy Balance

Energy balance obeys the laws of thermodynamics, especially the first law, which simply stated, says that "*Every natural process transforms energy and moves energy, but cannot create or eliminate it*".[2] From the standpoint of metabolic nutrition, we can further define energy balance as the state in which energy intake, in the form of food and/or alcohol, matches the energy expended through basal metabolism, the thermal effect of food (digestion), and physical activity" (Figure 1.5). If you are in energy balance, your weight will be stable and the amount of energy consumed will equal the amount of energy expended. If you don't eat, over time you will lose weight, and if you eat a lot more than you should, the energy will be stored, and over time you will gain weight. It's that simple.

The components of food–those macro- and micronutrients that you eat, drink, or take in through supplements constitute "energy intake", while basal metabolism, exercise, the thermal effect of food intake, and non-exercise thermogenesis constitute energy expenditure. Let's look at each of these components of energy intake and energy expenditure in more detail.

Food intake is regulated by complex signaling pathways that will be discussed later in this textbook. For the purpose of this discussion on energy balance, food intake simply constitutes the total number of calories taken in, whether it be from fat, carbohydrates, or proteins. The amount of energy that can be obtained from the food—usually at least 90% of the available energy in the food—is our energy intake. The remaining 10% is lost in the feces, urine, and respiration and simply not used

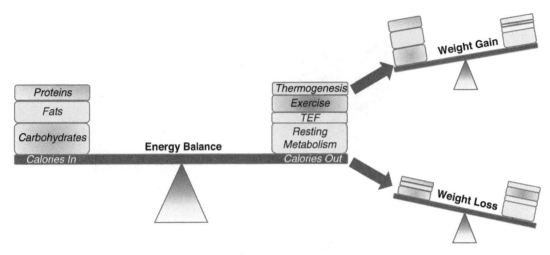

Figure 1.5: **Metabolic Energy Balance.** Obeying the First Law of thermodynamics, energy comes into the body in the form of food (and alcohol) and is expended by exercise, resting metabolism, thermogenesis, and the thermal effect of food (TEF). Energy can also be stored if intake exceeds energy use, and used when intake is less than energy needs.

as fuel[3]. The total available energy intake for an individual determines the total energy that individual has available, and whether energy will need to be stored, or burned for daily energy needs. While in a simple sense, the body tightly regulates hunger and energy needs, such that one would assume that energy balance would be the normal state. In reality, the physiological state of hunger, and the amount food and alcohol consumed, can also occur because of increased palpability of a food, as well as the context, or social and environmental situation in which food is present[4]. Thus, energy intake can exceed, or be less than, the energy needs for the organism.

As noted in Figure 1.5, energy expenditure can be divided into four main components—resting energy expenditure, thermal effect of food, thermogenesis, and active energy expenditure. The thermal effect of food (TEF) refers to the amount of energy that is required to digest the food into components that can be absorbed and stored. TEF can be different based on the type of food eaten-for example, while the TEF for an individual on a Western diet is about 10% of the total daily energy expenditure, the TEF can vary from 0–30% depending on the combination of proteins, fats, and carbohydrates consumed[5]. Protein requires the most energy to metabolize, followed by carbohydrates, and then fat. Why? Energetically these are more "expensive" to your energy budget because to make them into energy, energy has to be used.

Respiratory energy expenditure (REE) (also called resting metabolic rate—RMR), refers to the energy required for metabolism during rest; and according to one review, in sedentary individuals REE can account for up to 70% of total daily energy expenditure[4]. REE can be measured during sleep (sleep metabolic rate) or awake but in a restful state. When measured in an awake setting, REE is measured approximately 5% higher to maintain a wakeful state[4]. REE is influenced by

Our bacterial friends...or foes?

The bacteria in our guts can also harvest calories from food. Interestingly, in obese mice, the gut bacteria can actually harvest more calories from food than lean mice. This seems to be due to different types of bacteria that populate the guts of lean versus obese mice. Want to read more on this? Then take a look at this review article by Million and colleagues[5].

fat-free mass (your muscles, bones, organs, etc.), total fat mass, age, sex, genetics, and hormones, with fat free mass, age and sex accounting for up to 83% of the variance in non-obese, non-diabetic individuals[6].

The most variable component of energy expenditure is the contribution of activity, which occurs through the action of our muscles. This component of energy expenditure has both conscious or voluntary physical activity, and spontaneous or unconscious physical activity. Spontaneous physical activity includes things that you might not be conscious of, such as fidgeting, or just general twitches and movements, as well as the energy consumed to maintain posture. In 24-hour measurements, spontaneous activity could burn up to 700 kcals per day[7]. On the other hand, voluntary physical activity, which includes all of the things that we do during regular movement can be modulated by the individual. Swimming, running, walking, lifting weights, doing yoga—all of these can be considered voluntary physical activity. For sedentary individuals, activity-based energy expenditure might only contribute 15% of the total daily energy expenditure, while for very active individuals, up to 50% of energy can be burned by voluntary physical movement[4]. Thus, the more voluntary physical activity that you do on a daily basis, the more total energy you expend. Conversely, the more sedentary you are, the less total energy you expend, and if you want to maintain your current body weight, you might need to reduce calorie intake. Remember, food intake must balance energy expenditure to maintain body weight.

Finally, one last component in our energy expenditure category is facultative thermogenesis, which contributes to your total energy expenditure through the production of heat in response to environmental changes in temperature. We see this often in animals, who will show shivering in response to a cold temperature. Studies have shown that for every 1°C increase in body temperature that needs to be generated (i.e. in a cold environment), 10–15% more energy needs to be expended by the organism through increased facultative thermogenesis to maintain or raise body temperature and keep an individual warm[8]. While being cold is unpleasant, the reason the body maintains temperature within narrow limits is because the enzymes that run our metabolic reactions have been fine-tuned to work at 37°C. Facultative thermogenesis occurs in a tissue called brown fat, which we will talk about later in the textbook. Brown fat has been found in humans, but is found in much higher levels in animals than in humans[9].

> ### Did you know?
> When whole-body indirect calorimetry measures are made, proteins are not in the mix of what is being measured through the CO_2/O_2 levels-why? Because to measure protein metabolism one needs to look at urea, and blood levels of other metabolites. But we can still get very close to total energy expenditure measurements using just the CO_2/O_2 ratios with these calorimeters.

As we summarize this section on energy balance, realize that we are only briefly examining the contributions of each side of the equation (Figure 1.5) and that many cellular, molecular, and physiological processes can change or vary the contributions from "normal". However, it is important to have an initial view of what energy balance is, so that we can begin to think about what happens when it is disrupted.

Measuring Energy Balance-intake and Expenditure

Now that we know what energy balance is, and how it can be divided into intake and expenditure, we should consider how these are measured by scientists and physicians. There are several ways that we will discuss for each side of the equation, with advantages and disadvantages for each.

Determining the daily food intake in humans or experimental organisms ultimately considers the available energy in the food, and then calculates the total calorie intake over a 24-hour period. In mice, or other research animals, sophisticated balances hold food, and subtract the food that is eaten or taken from the balance. The researcher also needs to check the cage for any remaining food bits, but can use the weight of the food, and the known protein, fat, and carbohydrate content to calculate total daily energy intake. One can also take a slightly less sophisticated and more labor intensive approach, as we did in one of our intake studies[10], and simply measure the total amount of food in the bin, minus the amount gone from the bin the next day. Again, food crumbs in the bottom of the cage need to be accounted for, but even this slightly cruder method produces fairly consistent results.

While there are examples of giving human volunteers specific meals in a confined location so that total consumption can be measured similarly to rodents, measuring food intake in humans often means measuring their food intake in a free-roaming situation. In other words, many of the studies of human intake rely on the experimental subjects themselves providing their food intake through written or photographic food diaries[4]. These methods are standard in research studies, but can give confounding data due to the accuracy of self-report by volunteers and variability of food types[4], as compared to rodents where the intake is measured and food content is standardized. Another method used in some studies involves biomarkers, such as those for carbohydrates[11], to confirm reported intake. However, it is rare that this type of biomarker study is done in humans without additional dietary recall.

For energy expenditure, we have similar methods for measuring these in rodents or other experimental animals, and in humans. For rodents, the Comprehensive Lab Animal Monitoring System (CLAMS), such as that made by Columbus Instruments (Columbus, OH) incorporates environmentally-closed cages that measure respiration during rest, and physical activity to calculate total daily energy expenditure (Figure 1.6A). Physical activity can be further measured using X-Y-Z axis laser beam breaks, which allow the user determine if the animal is moving around the cage or resting in a single spot, for the calculation of resting or exercising energy expenditure. Food intake during the experiment can be measured using a balance, which weighs total amount of food remaining, giving the researcher the ability to assess total caloric intake during the experiment. Cages equipped with running wheels, allow scientists to measure voluntary energy expenditure in rodents (Figure 1.6B). These wheels have digital counters, with computer monitoring that allow one to measure total

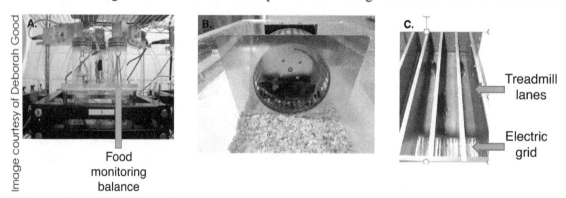

Image courtesy of Deborah Good

A.

B.

C.

Food monitoring balance

Treadmill lanes

Electric grid

Figure 1.6: **Equipment to Measure Food Intake and Energy Expenditure in Rodents.** (**A**) Metabolic cages. The cages are entirely enclosed so that air in/air out is measured (CO_2/O_2). Balances measure food and water intake, while laser beams measure X-Y-Z axis movement. (**B**) Rodent running wheels measure speed, total time, and total distance. Computer software allows for 24 hour exercise rhythms to be assessed. (**C**) Rodent treadmills can be programmed for different speeds, and inclines. Time running, before quitting is sured. Rodents who are no longer motivated to run will move to the electric grid and receive a small shock.

running distance during daytime and nighttime. The measurements are taken in increments so one can see when the animal is in its cage or on the wheel at any given time during the day. Finally, rodent treadmills for examining energy expenditure under forced conditions (Figure 1.6C). Treadmill apparatuses are most often separate from the home cage. Researchers place the rodent in a contained treadmill system and turn the treadmill on at a certain speed for a specified amount of time. The researcher can measure ability and motivation of the rodent to run during that time—any time the rodent stops running it will slip towards an electric grid which will administer a short shock once every three seconds. The rodent is then manually placed back on the treadmill by the researcher. If the rodent goes back to the electric grid and sits three times during a test, the rodent is usually removed from the treadmill and the time of removal recorded. Animals who have an inability or lack the motivation to run will have lower run times than those that are normal. In fact, normal rodents are known to run for 1 hour or more without ever sliding back to the shock grid! Some versions of the rodent treadmill can measure VCO_2/VO_2 during exercise, giving the added information on metabolism during exercise.

In humans, we also have several ways to measure energy expenditure (Figure 1.7). The first method uses a ventilated hood to measure REE, in which an individual lies down for about 30 minutes (in a fasted state), and carbon dioxide (CO_2) and metabolic oxygen (O_2) levels are measured (Figure 1.7A). Using ventilated hoods, resting energy expenditure can be measured very precisely to the calorie (kcal).

> **A calorie by any other name is still a calorie**
>
> The definition of a calorie (kcal) is the energy needed to raise 1 kilogram of water 1 degree Celsius.

Likewise, facemasks or mouth pieces can be used to measure energy expenditure during exercise, with a similar precision (Figure 1.7B). These methods are called indirect calorimetry because

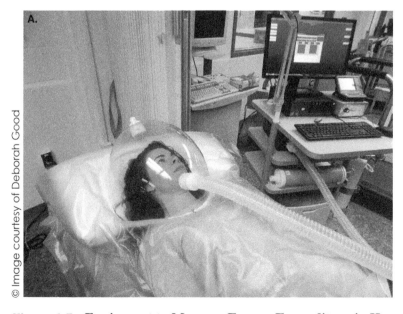
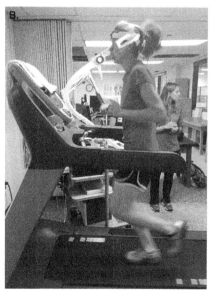

© Image courtesy of Deborah Good

Figure 1.7: Equipment to Measure Energy Expenditure in Humans via Indirect Calorimetry. (**A**) Resting energy expenditure can be measuring using a ventilated hood. The subject is recumbent and testing should occur at least 4 hours after their last meal. (**B**) $V\dot{O}_2$ is measured using a face mask worn while the subject is exercising, usually on a stationary bike or treadmill.

energy expenditure is calculated indirectly from the amount of oxygen consumption and carbon dioxide production. Oxygen is needed for metabolism and carbon dioxide is the byproduct of macromolecule catabolism. By measuring the consumption and production of these gases, one indirectly determines the amount of metabolism going on. In a second method, individuals are placed in a room, called a "whole room calorimeter" and the individual's energy expenditure is measured during an entire 24-hour period (can be direct or indirect calorimetry). That means that energy expenditure during rest, sleep, while eating, and during exercise can be precisely measured, also by assessing oxygen consumed and carbon dioxide produced (indirect) or by assessing heat produced (direct). This is similar to the CLAMS systems described for rodents. The total fat and carbohydrate utilization (down to the gram level) can be measured using whole room calorimetry. The final type of energy expenditure method presented, utilizes doubly-labeled water. In this procedure, regular drinking water that contains stably-labeled radioisotopes on hydrogen and oxygen, and when a person drinks this water, it equilibrates with the water in their body. The rate at which the metabolites that contain radio-labeled hydrogen and oxygen show up in your breath, sweat, and urine correlates to their metabolic rate. For all of the methods described, the procedures are generally not done in a doctor's office, but rather, are research methods, and performed by scientists studying metabolism.

Finally, researchers often want to know the lean and fat mass percentages of an individual for comparison of REE, and exercise levels. There are measures for this in both rodents and humans (Figure 1.8). In humans, dual-energy x-ray absorptiometry or DEXA analysis, is one of the ways used to measure the total amount of fat versus lean tissue in an individual (Figure 1.8A). It is based on a three-compartment model: bone, fat mass, and lean mass. This is the same machine that hospitals use to measure bone mineral density, but it also measures body fat and lean mass. Since lean mass is one of the greatest contributors to REE, and body fat represents stored energy, this measurement is also very important when considering both food intake and energy expenditure in humans as well as rodents. Individuals can also do anthropometric measurements to assess body proportions. Using height and weight to do a simple body mass index (BMI) calculation is an example of a height-weight index that can be compared to societal weight standards. Assessing abdominal fat can be done with a hip-to-waist ratio and comparing the ratio to healthy standards: <0.8 for women and <0.9 for men. Both of these will provide some data on whether the individual can be considered normal weight, underweight, overweight, or obese. Calipers, when used correctly, can measure body fat with just a 3% +/- accuracy rate (Figure 1.8B). For rodents, a rodent-sized magnetic resonance imaging (MRI) machine uses mathematical density calculations to get total body fat calculations and lean mass calculations for both normal and obese rodents (Figure 1.8C). In this figure, the fat is colored in light blue and one can see much more of it in the genetically obese rodent, when compared to the normal rodent. Many individual labs that study metabolism have access to a rodent body fat analyzer, which is based on nuclear magnetic resonance (NMR) (Figure 1.8D). The machine gathers proton signals during a specific period of time, and based on the body weight of the rodent, provides the researchers with lean mass, fat mass, and total water in the rodent. Together and separately, these pieces of equipment can give precise information on body fat levels in humans and animals.

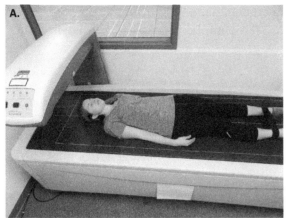
© Image courtesy of Deborah Good

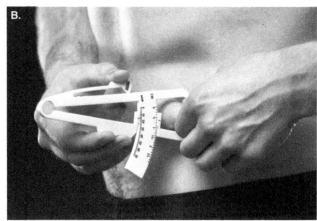
© luckyraccoon/Shutterstock.com

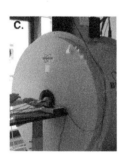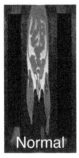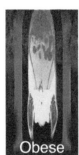
Normal   Obese
© Image courtesy of Deborah Good

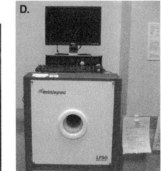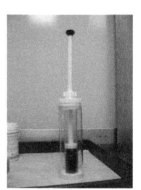
© Image courtesy of Deborah Good

Figure 1.8: Equipment to Measure Body Fat and Lean Mass in Humans and Rodents. (A) A DEXA machine measures lean and fat body mass in a recumbent individual. **(B)** Skin fold measurements, using calipers can estimate body fat levels in humans and other animals. **(C)** Rodent MRI machines can gather whole body information from rodents. The rodents must be anesthetized so as not to move during this procedure **(D)** Nuclear Magnetic Resonance (NMR) is used to gather lean and fat mass information from non-anesthetized rodents. The rodents are placed in the tube for less than one minute at a time to get the information, and calculations based on body weight give body composition data.

Summary

As we end this first chapter, you should think about the various contributions to metabolism in an individual, including the composition of food taken into the body, the amount of energy expended by the individual, as well as environmental, genetic, and even behavioral or social differences in that individual. In the more "normal" situation, energy intake is balanced with energy expenditure and weight is stable. We will discuss the "abnormal" situations later in the text, both where energy intake is in excess over expenditure, and the opposite—where energy intake is low and cannot supply sufficient calories for all the metabolic and exercise energy demands. These two latter situations will cause the systems in the body to shift fuel sources and change metabolic needs when possible. The end goal for any individual's body is to maintain essential metabolic processes and sustain life.

Points to Ponder

➤ Does eating sugar and/or fat *cause* weight gain, independent of energy balance? If you said yes, how? If you said no, why not? Consider coming back to this question after later chapters.

➤ Are low carbohydrate diets better than low fat diets? What is the macronutrient composition of both, and why or why not might one diet work better than others? Would genetics play a role?

➤ Is exercise important for weight loss? How does your exercise level contribute to total energy expenditure? What other factors contribute?

References

1. Alpert T, Herzel L, Neugebauer KM. Perfect timing: splicing and transcription rates in living cells. *Wiley Interdiscip Rev RNA*. 2017;8(2).
2. First Law of Thermodynamics. https://www.allaboutscience.org/first-law-of-thermodynamics-faq.htm. Accessed January 31, 2018.
3. Widdowson EM. Assessment of the energy value of human foods. *Proc Nutr Soc*. 1955;14(2):142–154.
4. Lam YY, Ravussin E. Analysis of energy metabolism in humans: A review of methodologies. *Mol Metab*. 2016;5(11):1057–1071.
5. Million M, Lagier JC, Yahav D, Paul M. Gut bacterial microbiota and obesity. *Clin Microbiol Infect*. 2013;19(4):305–313.
6. Bogardus C, Lillioja S, Ravussin E, et al. Familial dependence of the resting metabolic rate. *N Engl J Med*. 1986;315(2):96–100.
7. Weyer C, Snitker S, Rising R, Bogardus C, Ravussin E. Determinants of energy expenditure and fuel utilization in man: effects of body composition, age, sex, ethnicity and glucose tolerance in 916 subjects. *Int J Obes Relat Metab Disord*. 1999;23(7):715–722.
8. Landsberg L. Core temperature: a forgotten variable in energy expenditure and obesity? *Obes Rev*. 2012;13 Suppl 2:97–104.
9. Cohen P, Spiegelman BM. Brown and Beige Fat: Molecular Parts of a Thermogenic Machine. *Diabetes*. 2015;64(7):2346–2351.
10. Coyle CA, Strand SC, Good DJ. Reduced activity without hyperphagia contributes to obesity in Tubby mutant mice. *Physiol Behav*. 2008;95(1–2):168–175.
11. Tasevska N. Urinary Sugars--A Biomarker of Total Sugars Intake. *Nutrients*. 2015;7(7):5816–5833.

Energy!

Introduction

Being in energy balance is modulated by the calorie input (influenced by hunger and satiety, as well as the environment), and the calorie output (influenced by energy expenditure) for the individual. Remaining in energy balance is really an individual process—each of us are genetically, environmentally, socially, and physiologically different and will have different metabolic needs. The book as a whole, will focus on this topic extensively, so this paragraph will be brief. Your energy balance, and perturbations to your energy balance ultimately affect your weight, especially over the long-term—it's the first law of the laws of thermodynamics, as discussed in the first chapter. As a reminder, the first law of thermodynamics, which is also known as the Law of the Conservation of Energy, states in the simplest terms that energy cannot be created or destroyed in an isolated system. We can extend this a bit, to think about the fact that in the closed and isolated system of our bodies, energy can change forms (i.e. making ATP from food), and can flow from one place to another (i.e. using energy or storing it). So, what does this mean for human (and other animals') energy balance? This law of thermodynamics exemplifies the "energy in = energy out" theory that we will discuss throughout the book. Let's start by defining what cellular energy is, and how we can make it in the body.

What is satiety?

Most define satiety as the state of being fed to, or beyond capacity. So, think about that last big meal you had, and you'll get the idea!

Adenosine Tri-Phosphate

As introduced in chapter 1, Adenosine Tri-Phosphate (ATP) is the key molecule to consider for energy that is produced or used in our cells. Energy is stored in phosphate bonds within the ATP molecule. When one of these bonds is used for a metabolic reaction, the molecule loses a phosphate group and becomes adenosine Di-phosphate (ADP) (Figure 2.1). The last phosphate group—that which has the gamma bond (γ) is the one that is hydrolyzed. There is also a form called adenosine Mono-phosphate (AMP) where the beta bond (β) has been hydrolyzed leaving one phosphate group remaining, but the main molecules cycling for our energy processes occurs between ATP and ADP, which hold onto, or move phosphates from one molecule to another using the hydrolysis and reformation of the γ–bond to do so. There are a couple of reactions that we'll talk about later that actually cleave the β–bond from ATP to AMP in one step, resulting in the production of AMP and a pyro-phosphate (P_i-P_i), but this is a much rarer reaction.

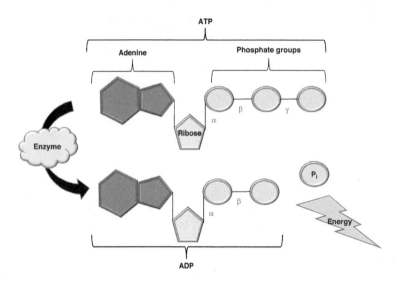

Figure 2.1: **Adenosine Tri- and Di-phosphate.** Both Adenosine tri-phosphate (ATP) and adenosine di-phosphate (ADP) are composed of an adenine and ribose backbone with phosphate groups. The key difference is the number of phosphate groups available. ATP has stored energy, with the highest level of energy available in its gamma (γ) bond.

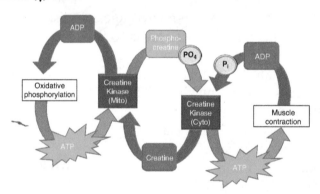

Figure 2.2: **The Creatine Phosphate System.** Oxidative phosphorylation within mitochondria creates ATP, and this ATP can transfer a phosphate to be stored on creatine, generating creatine phosphate (or phosphocreatine). The mitochondrial creatine kinase molecule performs this reaction. Phosphocreatine can migrate to the cytoplasm where muscular contraction is taking place. Within the cytoplasm creatine kinase can work to transfer the stored phosphate from phosphocreatine to ADP making ATP. This cytoplasmic ATP can now be used to do cellular work, such as muscle contraction.

Lots of proteins (enzymes) can interact with and use ATP, but one of these proteins, creatine can hold onto and "store" phosphates (P_i), especially within our muscle, for quick ATP generation. As shown in Figure 2.2, two forms of the enzyme creatine kinase shuttle phosphates between creatine and phosphocreatine (also called creatine phosphate) within the mitochondrial and cytoplasmic compartments of the cell. Phosphocreatine is an energy reserve, and the reaction performed by creatine kinase can go in both directions—either creating phosphocreatine or releasing the phosphate group to create ATP leaving unphosphorylated creatine.

Do you supplement?

Many people have used creatine supplements. You can find large jars of this protein on the shelves of grocery and health-food stores. Is there evidence that creatine supplement is effective? YES! But only in certain types of situations. Read on in the text for more information.

Creatine supplementation does increase phosphocreatine levels in skeletal muscle, and this added phosphocreatine can be important when an individual engages in short-term, high intensity exercise[1,2]. It is hypothesized that when creatine is ingested during rest, the levels of phosphocreatine are replenished in skeletal muscle, translating into a higher or improved performance when the individual participates in high intensity exercise (exercises that last 10–15 sec.). Think of this as a little energy bar for our muscles. For example, in a recent meta-analysis which looked at 53 studies, including over 500 individuals that had either creatine supplementation or were not supplemented, the overall conclusion was that those who received supplementation had a higher upper limb performance, (i.e. for bench press) but this effect only lasted 3 minutes over those that did not receive supplementation[3]. The same group found that supplementation could also improve lower limb performance (squat and leg press), again with only a 3-minute duration over those not being supplemented[4]. Some caveats of these findings (and many others in the literature) include—there are many different regimens for supplementation, long-term effects of supplementation are not known, and that while creatine is generally thought to be safe, the safety of supplementing in children or adolescent individuals has not been rigorously studied[5]. It is important to note that creatine is a nitrogen containing organic acid and as such, high supplementation intakes may overburden the liver and the kidneys. Supplementation should always follow recommended daily amounts.

Making ATP

Creatine kinase's utilization of phosphocreatine to add a phosphate to ADP making ATP is an example of substrate-level phosphorylation. In substrate-level phosphorylation, the γ phosphate group from ATP is transferred to another protein (Figure 2.3). For phosphocreatine, this is a production reaction that is also used for storage of the high energy phosphate bond. Any time a phosphate group is transferred from one protein to another, with enzymatic production of ATP, we have substrate-level phosphorylation. As we will see later, two enzymes of glycolysis and one enzyme of the TriCarboxylic Acid (TCA) cycle also perform substrate-level phosphorylation. By doing so, these enzymes create ATP molecules for use in other energy-demanding reactions.

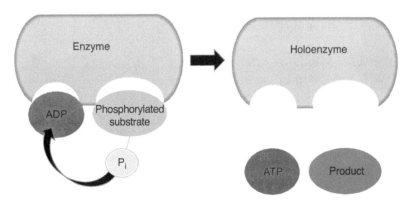

Figure 2.3: **Substrate Level Phosphorylation.** Enzymes (such as creatine kinase and those found in glycolysis) will take the phosphate group from a phosphorylated substrate and transfer it to ADP, forming ATP and the unphosphorylated product. An enzyme that has completed it's enzymatic reaction and is ready for the next is called a "holoenzyme."

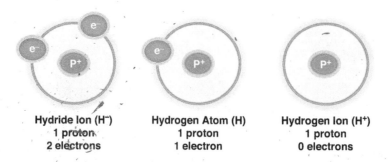

Hydride Ion (H⁻)
1 proton
2 electrons

Hydrogen Atom (H)
1 proton
1 electron

Hydrogen Ion (H⁺)
1 proton
0 electrons

Figure 2.4: **The Multiple States of Hydrogen.** The hydride ion (H⁻) can donate electrons, while the hydrogen ion (H⁺) can receive them.

Before proceeding very far into this, we need to step back and talk about oxidation and reduction reactions, in which electrons are donated and accepted. You must have both in a reaction—one substrate donating electrons and one accepting electrons for the reaction to proceed. There are specific names for these—the oxidizer donates electrons (LEO- loses electron oxidation), while the reducing substrate gains electrons (GER- gains electron reduction). That might seem counterintuitive, but consider that the reduced substrate will gain electrons, which are negatively charged, and reduce in overall charge, due to that change. Thus, oxidation is the loss of electrons, and an increase in overall charge to the substrate.

Electron movement in substrates occurs via proton movement—yes, the protons or H⁺ molecules are the ones that are moving through the system. Hydrogen can come in several "flavors" (Figure 2.4)—the hydrogen atom, which has one proton and one electron, the hydride ion, which has one proton and two electrons, and a charge of (-), and the hydrogen ion, which has one proton and no electrons, or a charge of (+). These hydrogens are located on co-enzymatic molecules (many times these are vitamins and minerals, and you'll learn more about them in the accompanying textbook on micronutrients), or on the substrates in the reaction.

Let's take a look as some of these reactions, which are termed "redox reactions" (Figure 2.5). Coenzymes such as nicotinamide dinucleotide (NAD⁺, or the vitamin B3, **Figure 2.5A**), or Flavin dinucleotide (FAD⁺, or the vitamin B2, **Figure 2.5B**), participate in these redox reactions. NAD⁺ and nicotinamide adenine dinucleotide phosphate (NADP⁺) can each accept a hydride ion (H:⁻), becoming NADH and NADPH, respectively, with a H⁺ released into solution. These can be oxidized by donating an H:⁻. Likewise, FAD⁺ is reduced, and can accept two hydrogen ions to become $FADH_2$. $FADH_2$ can be oxidized by donating two hydrogen ions to a reaction.

Many of these redox reactions—and especially those creating ATP will occur within the mitochondria (Figure 2.6). Mitochondria coordinate oxidation of carbohydrates (sugars), fats, and to a lesser extent, proteins. Mitochondria perform this cellular function using mitochondrial proteins, some of which are produced from the mitochondrial genome, and some of which are produced by the nuclear DNA and transported into the mitochondria. Mitochondria are shaped (somewhat) like a kidney bean, at least from electron microscopy studies that can visualize the ultra-structure of the mitochondria, including the cristae, or inner membrane

> **Fun fact**
>
> A transcription factor, TFAM, which is required for transcription of mitochondria DNA during mitochondrial biogenesis (duplication) is actually encoded by a nuclear gene. Thus, while it is hypothesized that mitochondria might have evolved from an independent organism, mitochondria and the cells they live in are now completely dependent on each other.

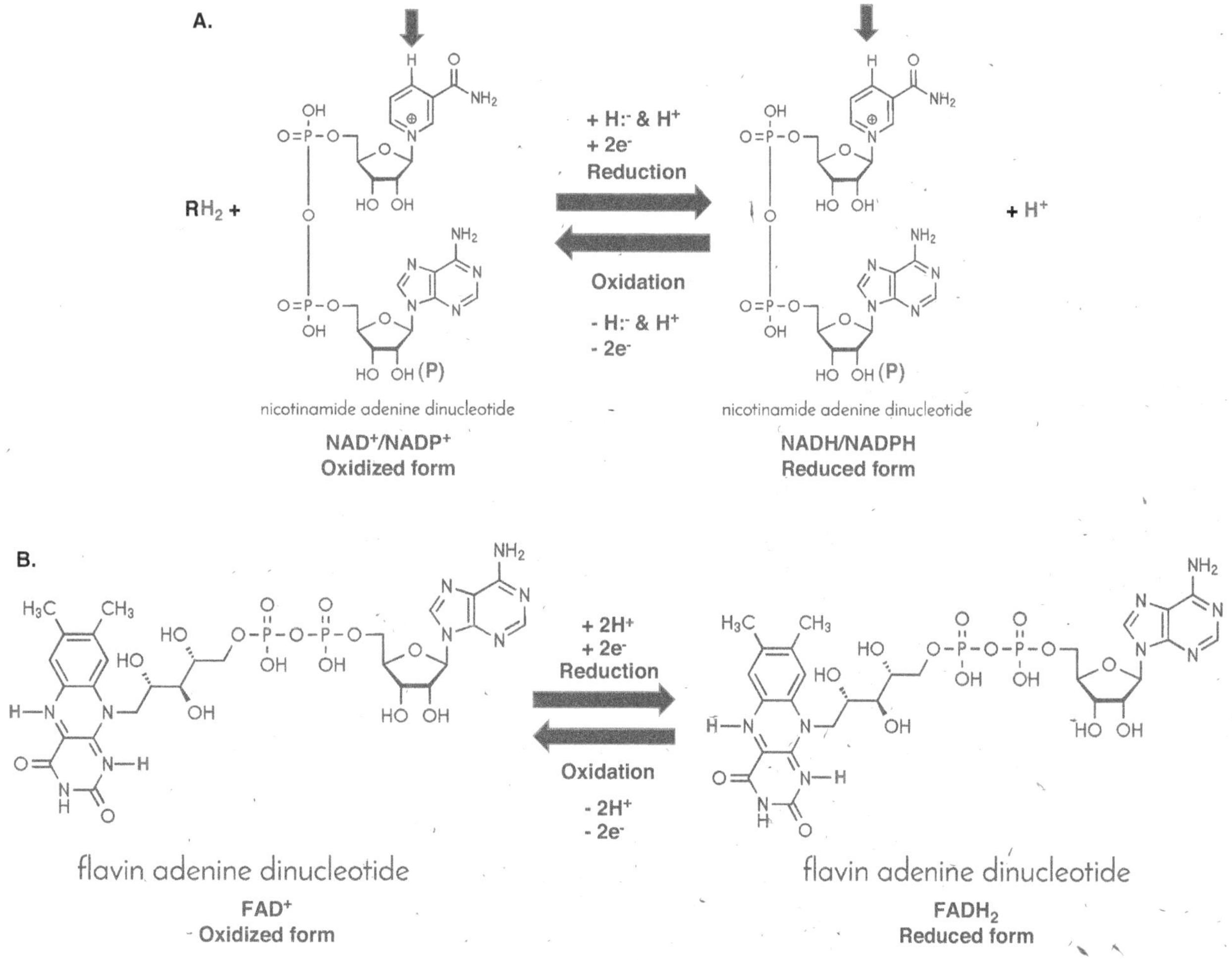

A.

$RH_2 +$

+ H:⁻ & H⁺
+ 2e⁻
Reduction

Oxidation

- H:⁻ & H⁺
- 2e⁻

+ H⁺

nicotinamide adenine dinucleotide
NAD⁺/NADP⁺
Oxidized form

nicotinamide adenine dinucleotide
NADH/NADPH
Reduced form

B.

+ 2H⁺
+ 2e⁻
Reduction

Oxidation

- 2H⁺
- 2e⁻

flavin adenine dinucleotide
FAD⁺
Oxidized form

flavin adenine dinucleotide
FADH₂
Reduced form

Figure 2.5: **Co-enzymatic Oxidation and Reduction Reactions.** The two most common oxidation/ reduction reactions occur with (**A**) nicotinamide adenine dinucleotide (NAD⁺/NADP⁺ in its oxidized form and NADH/NADPH in its reduced form) and (**B**) Flavin adenine dinucletide (FAD⁺ in its oxidized form, and FADH₂ in its reduced form).

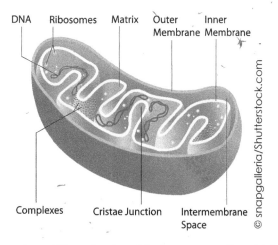

Figure 2.6: **Mitochondrial Structure.** The mitochondria is an organelle which has both an inner and outer membrane (and you'll see why this is important later), and its own DNA (mtDNA) as well as ribosomes floating around in the mitochondrial matrix

which is highly folded and densely packed. Mitochondria also contain, as mentioned before, its own DNA (mtDNA), which unlike nuclear DNA that is packed into chromosomes, is circular, in multiple copies, and only contains 13 protein coding genes. Finally, there is an outer membrane that has porin proteins—which can allow molecules less than 50 kilodalton (kDa) to pass through into the mitochondria. It was originally thought that these pores would allow for pyruvate (the product of glycolysis) and some proteins to come into the mitochondria, and waste (ex. CO_2) and ATP to come out of the mitochondria. However, recent work has identified a mitochondria pyruvate transporter[3], and there has been renewed interest with some contradicting evidence in an adenine transporter that seems to transfer ATP out, and ADP into the mitochondria[6,7]. Other larger molecules like long chain fatty acids, use a carrier system (carnitine shuttle) to enter the mitochondria.

It is in the mitochondria that oxidative phosphorylation, where substrates (i.e. our fats, carbohydrates, and proteins), are converted into energy (Figure 2.7). We will spend a lot of time on these processes in this textbook, so this section is meant only to introduce the topic.

Ratios of ATP/ADP and NADH/NAD$^+$ are indicative of the energy status of the cell. This is key to metabolic regulation. A high ATP/ADP ratio (i.e. when ATP levels are higher than ADP) means that energy demands are generally being met, and no additional ATP needs to be made. Alternatively, a low ATP/ADP ratio means the opposite—the cell is in a state of deficit, and needs to make more ATP. This suggests that there is an increase in energy demand. The higher amount of ADP signals to the cell that ATP needs to be made to compensate for the increased energy demand. Similarly, the NADH/NAD$^+$ ratio also is a measure of energy demand. A lower NADH/NAD$^+$ ratio means that NADH is being oxidized to NAD$^+$, and there is a need for more ATP. Conversely, a high NADH/NAD$^+$ ratio suggest that energy demands are likely being met.

As an example of how these ratios can be considered, using real life situations, what happens when you stand up? Energy demands go up—right? So, the ATP/ADP ratio would be lower, indicating the need to make more ATP. The NADH/NAD$^+$ ratio will be low—again indicating that NADH is being used in ATP-generating reactions (ex. donating electrons to the electron transport

> **Consider this**
>
> ...Can you think of other situations that might affect ATP/ADP and NADH/NAD$^+$ ratios?

chain). How about when you are running, and then finish the race and stop? In this case, the ATP/ADP ratio would have been low, but then would switch to being higher, as your energy demands decrease when stopped and resting. Likewise, the NADH/NAD$^+$ ratio would have been lower as well, and then would switch to being higher, as demands are being met.

Macronutrient Oxidation

All of these examples of ATP/ADP and NADH/NAD$^+$ ratios rely on changes in macronutrient oxidation, or the breakdown (oxidation) of glucose, fatty acids, ketones, and the carbon skeletons of proteins (Figure 2.7). In brief (as we will spend much more time on this in later chapters), glucose oxidation occurs in the cytoplasm (a.k.a., cytosol) of the cells, in a stepwise process called glycolysis, ending with the production of 2 pyruvate, 2 ATP, and 2 NADH, in aerobic conditions. Pyruvate can then enter the mitochondria, and be converted to acetyl CoA. Acetyl CoA can now enter the TCA cycle. Fats go through a different process called beta-oxidation, producing 1 NADH and 1 $FADH_2$ each cycle, which can feed directly into the electron transport cycle. Each cycle removes two carbons from the fatty acid chain, producing an acetyl CoA that then feeds into the TCA cycle.

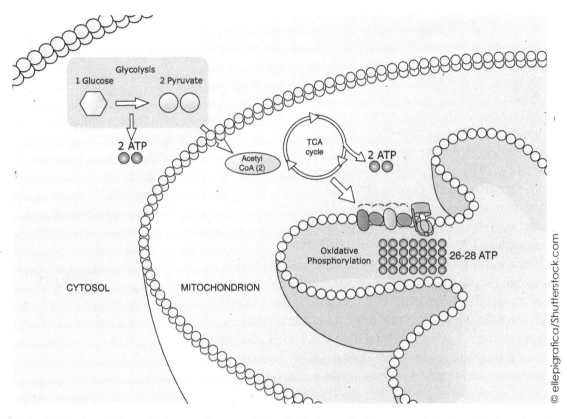

Figure 2.7: **Mitochondria—the Powerhouse of the Cell.** Glycolysis can produce two ATP molecules, but the real powerhouse of the cell is the mitochondria, where the TCA produces two more ATP, and feeds electrons carried by NADH and $FADH_2$ to the electron transport cycle. There, oxidative phosphorylation converts these to 28 (slow oxidative muscle) or 26 (fast glycolytic muscle) ATP molecules for use in other energy-requiring reactions in the cell, for an overall ATP production for one molecule of glucose of 32 ATP in slow oxidative muscle or 30 ATP in fast oxidative muscle.

Beta oxidation occurs within the mitochondria. The carbon backbones of ketogenic amino acids (stripped of their nitrogen) can also be broken down, resulting in the production of acetyl CoA that can feed into the TCA cycle. Proteins, as we will see in later chapters have additional entries into different parts of the TCA cycle, in addition to acetyl CoA. (The carbon backbones of glucogenic amino acids can be used to make pyruvate and other TCA cycle intermediates.) The common denominator though, for proteins, fats, and carbohydrates is to enter the TCA cycle as acetyl CoA. The TCA cycle is a cyclic process which takes acetyl CoA and combines it with oxaloacetate converting it to citrate, then isocitrate and so on, through a series oxidative dehydration reactions producing electrons that can flow into the electron transfer chain (ETC) by way of NADH and $FADH_2$. The ETC, with the ultimate ending enzyme ATP synthase, produces ATP which can be used for all of the other energy-requiring metabolic reactions in our bodies. Let's talk more about oxidative phosphorylation and the upstream TCA cycle.

Did you know?

In biochemistry, the words *synthetase* and *synthase*, in imply two different types of enzymes. Synthetases combine molecules (acting as a ligase) to make new molecules). Synthetases usually *use* ATP, as the process requires energy. Synthases on the other hand break chemical bonds to produce new molecules, and require much less energy. Now does it make sense why ATP Synthase is a synthase and not a synthetase?

The TCA Cycle

The TCA cycle is also known as the citric acid cycle, and the Krebs cycle (Figure 2.8). The TCA cycle goes in one direction, from acetyl CoA through multiple products/substrates, to produce 2 molecules of CO_2 (which we mostly exhale), 3 molecules of NADH, one molecule of $FADH_2$, and one GTP (which can be pretty quickly converted to ATP). The NADH and $FADH_2$ molecules are then shuttled to the electron transport chain to ultimately produce ATP for use in other reactions.

> **Moments in History**
>
> The Krebs Cycle, which we refer to as the TCA cycle, was named after German-Born physician and biochemist, Sir Hans Adolf Krebs, who received the Nobel prize in 1953, sharing it with Fritz Albert Lipmann, who discovered coenzyme A[8].

For one turn of the TCA cycle, with reducing equivalents (NADH and $FADH_2$) going to the ETC, 10 ATP molecules can be produced. This is because each NADH results in a maximum of 2.5 ATP (so three NADH from the TCA, entering into the ETC equals 7.5 ATP produced); each $FADH_2$ results in a maximum of 1.5 ATP per molecule (so add in another 1.5 ATP molecules produced) and the GTP can be used to form 1 ATP. The total then made is 10. Not bad right?

Let's dig a little deeper into the TCA cycle by looking at the individual reactions. Overall, the concentrations of the substrate and products on each side of each reaction can drive the TCA cycle, which is only going in one direction. There are 3 non-equilibrium reactions that are important regulatory steps. In other words, the direction of the cycle overall, and the products being produced can feedback and slow down, or speed up the reactions. The 3 non-equilibrium reactions are citrate

> **What do you think?**
>
> What happens in a person with osteoporosis, where calcium levels might be low? Would this affect overall energy productions?

synthase, isocitrate dehydrogenase, and α-ketoglutarate dehydrogenase. The first non-equilibrium regulatory step we are going to discuss involves the production of citrate from oxaloacetate and the incoming acetyl CoA via the enzyme citrate synthase. NADH is a negative allosteric inhibitor attaching to citrate synthase and, at least for the enzyme from *E. coli* that was used for conformational studies, binding of NADH changes its shape[9] (see Figure 2.8). Actually, NADH is also a negative allosteric regulator of the other two non-equilibrium reactions (isocitrate dehydrogenase and α-ketoglutarate dehydrogenase) too. Think about this for a minute, if NADH is high this signifies that energy (ATP) demands are likely being met, thus we can slow down the TCA cycle at multiple points because we do not need to be making more ATP. Likewise, the product of the citrate synthase reaction, citrate, is a competitive inhibitor for oxaloacetate—in other words, if there is a buildup of citrate, oxaloacetate cannot bind to citrate synthase, slowing down or stopping the reaction. Calcium is an overall positive allosteric regulator of the TCA cycle as it will increase activity of both isocitrate dehydrogenase and α-ketoglutarate dehydrogenase[10]. In other words, increased calcium signals high energy demands (especially in muscle where calcium stores are released in preparation for contraction), leading to increased activity of both enzymes. Why does this occur? Unlike the allosteric inhibitors discussed for citrate synthase, calcium actually serves as a regulatory structural co-factor for the mitochondrial dehydrogenases, being required for the overall activity and structure of the enzyme[11]. Succinyl CoA, which is the product the α-ketoglutarate dehydrogenase also serves as a competitive inhibitor of CoA for this reaction, just like we discussed above for oxaloacetate competitive inhibition of citrate synthase. Take a minute to think about this too, if succinyl CoA is

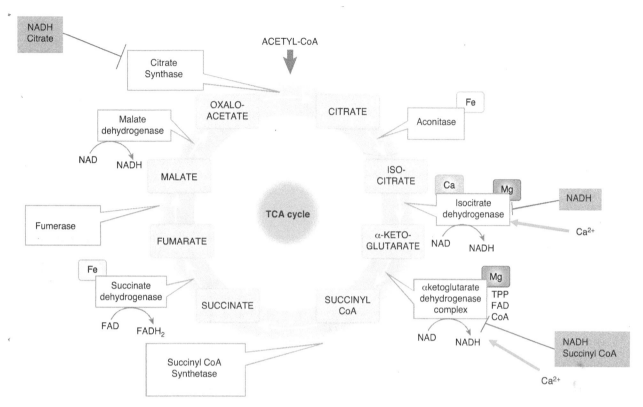

Figure 2.8: **The TCA Cycle.** The substrate/intermediates are shown in purple boxes, while the enzymes are listed in blue boxes. Note the enzymatic reactions that produce NADH and FADH$_2$. Inhibitors of the non-equilibrium reactions (either competively or allosterically) are shown in red and allosteric activators are shown in green.

accumulating more does not need to be made, thus **α**-ketoglutarate dehydrogenase should be slowed down to reduce further production. Other key reactions are those producing energy including the reaction catalyzed by succinate dehydrogenase, which produces one FADH$_2$ molecule, and is interesting in that this enzyme is also integral to complex 2 of the ETC, which will be discussed on more detail later. Finally, the reaction catalyzed by malate dehydrogenase produces an NADH to feed into the electron transport chain.

The Electron Transport Chain

The Electron Transport Chain (ETC) consists of four enzyme complexes along with ATP Synthase. All of these are embedded into the inner mitochondrial membrane. The reactions occurring in the ETC are oxidation-reduction reactions—essentially, electrons are being passed from NADH and FADH$_2$, which were generated in the TCA cycle or glycolysis, through complexes 1–4 (Figure 2.9). These reactions generate energy which is then used to pump protons (hydrogen ions) from the mitochondrial matrix to the intermembrane space against their gradient. In the last step of the ETC, the electrons are added to an oxygen molecule, forming water. Overall, the protons become more concentrated in the intermembrane space, as compared to the mitochondrial matrix. ATP Synthase uses the flow of these protons down their gradient to provide the energy to phosphorylate ADP, producing ATP. Proton pumping is integral to the entire concept of oxidative

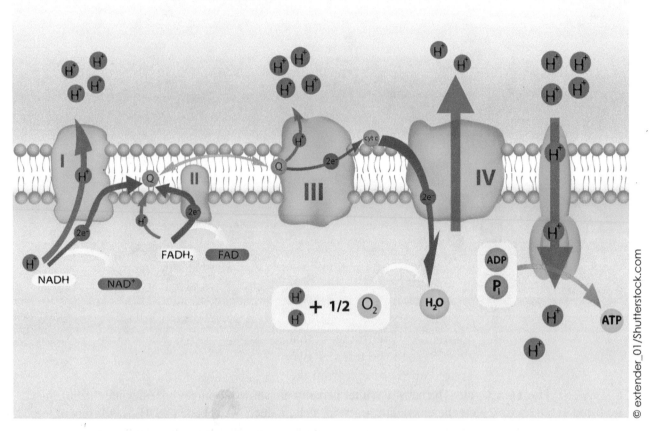

© extender_01/Shutterstock.com

Figure 2.9: **The Electron Transport Chain.** Four complexes, along with ATP Synthase make up the electron transport chain. Note the flow of H+ (protons), and the reductions of NADH, and $FADH_2$ through the complexes.

phosphorylation, and the inner and outer membranes of the mitochondria allow for proton pumping and formation of an electro-chemical gradient which is integral to energy production. ATP synthase uses that gradient to produce ATP.

Chemiosmotic Theory for ATP Production

The chemiosmotic theory for ATP Production states that there is a connection between electron transfer and the formation of ATP. Dr. Peter Dennis Mitchell who lived from September 29, 1920 and April 10, 1992, received the Nobel Prize in 1978 "for his contribution to the understanding of biological energy transfer through the formulation of the chemiosmotic theory"[12].

The differential gradient of protons between in intermembrane space where they are higher, and the matrix where the protons are lower results in an electrochemical gradient. There is a differential pH between the two

> **Of note**
>
> When one says "low" protons or "low" pH in these systems, this doesn't mean crazy low, such as a pH of 1.0—everything stays within physiological limits but are low or high enough to establish a gradient between the two systems, in this case the inner and outer mitochondrial membrane.

compartments as well as a differential charge between the two compartments. The pH in the intermembrane space is lower (i.e. more acidic, due to more protons) as compared to the pH in the matrix (i.e. more basic, due to fewer protons) and the intermembrane space is more positive (i.e. protons are positive) compared to the matrix. It is essential to have this polarized electrochemical gradient to product ATP. As shown in Figure 2.9, protons are pumped into the intermembrane space, against a gradient (because there are already more protons in that area), during electron transfer down the chain and where electrons finally combine with oxygen. The return of protons through ATP synthase releases energy. One way to think about this is that there is a higher gradient in the intermembrane space, and when that higher proton load is used to relieve some of the pressures in that area, energy can be released. A good analogy to this is a dam that is used to generate kinetic energy by water flowing and turning turbines to produce electricity. Likewise, flow of the protons back to the matrix results in turning of the "turbines" in the enzyme ATP Synthase, leading to energy production.

As noted above, each of the complexes in the ETC are composed of multiple proteins that function together as an enzyme complex. NADH-Coenzyme Q Oxidoreductase, otherwise known as Complex I is the first of these. This complex has 42 protein subunits, with 35 of these encoded by nuclear genes, and 7 encoded by mitochondrial DNA (Table 2.1). The proteins that make up Complex I work together to the transfer two electrons from the NADH molecules coming from the TCA cycle, as well as others sources such as glycolysis, pyruvate oxidation, and beta oxidation, both to be

discussed in detail later, to generate enough energy to pump four protons into the intermembrane space. Complex II, or Succinate Coenzyme Q Oxidoreductase (a.k.a., succinate dehydrogenase) is composed of four protein subunits, and all four of these are encoded by the nucleus (no mitochondrial genes). Do you remember succinate dehydrogenase from the TCA cycle? You should, as this enzyme complex serves TCA and ETC reactions. While there is not sufficient energy to pump protons at this step, this complex does reduce coenzyme Q to QH_2. Complex III or Coenzyme Q Cytochrome C Oxidoreductase has 11 protein parts—10 of which are encoded by nuclear genes, and one by a mitochondrial gene. In this complex, cytochrome C accepts one electron from QH_2. Thus, to get each electron into the ETC, you need two cytochrome C molecules. Each will generate sufficient energy to pump 4 protons across into the intermembrane space. The final complex in the ETC

Table 2.1: Electron Transport Chain Complexes, and ATP Synthase are made using nuclear and mitochondrial genes.

Complex	Protein subunits	Mitochondrial Genes	Nuclear Genes
Complex I/NADH Dehydrogenase Complex	42 proteins	7 genes	35 genes
Complex II/Succinate Coenzyme Q Oxidoreductase	4 proteins	0 genes	4 genes
Complex III/Coenzyme Q Cytochrome C Oxidoreductase	11 proteins	1 gene	10 genes
Complex IV/Cytochrome C Oxidase	13 proteins	3 genes	10 genes
ATP Synthase	20 proteins	2 genes	18 genes

is Cytochrome C Oxidase, or Complex IV. This complex is composed of 13 protein subunits, three of which are from mitochondrial genes, and 10 from nuclear genes. As the final step in the process, electrons are passed and sufficient energy is produced to pump two more electrons to the intermembrane space. At the end of this process, water is produced, as can be simply seen using the equation:

$$O_2 + 4e^- + 4H^+ \rightarrow 2H_2O$$

Unlike the TCA cycle where there are multiple "control points" within the cycle, the only known control point for the ETC is ATP demand (while there are probably more yet to be discovered). If ATP demand goes up, the flow through the ETC cycle will go up. Likewise, as ATP levels go up (and demand goes down), the ETC flow will slow down. This depends on regulation of ATP synthase. So, let's talk about ATP Synthase, which is not officially part of the ETC but is the final enzyme complex in the process of making ATP.

As shown in Figure 2.10, part of the structure of ATP Synthase does indeed look like a turbine. The enzyme is composed of two subunits (F_0 and F_1), made up of 20 proteins, with only two of these protein-coding genes encoded by the mitochondrial genome and the rest by the nuclear genome (Table 2.1). As H^+ pass through the c subunits of F_0, a rotation of the turbine-like subunit is created that is transferred to the γ subunit, which is in turn rotated relative to the β subunit or nucleotide subunit, which causes ADP to be phosphorylated. Per pair of electrons transferred from NADH eventually to oxygen, 10 protons are pumped from the matrix to the outer membrane space. $FADH_2$ electrons result in 6 protons pumped from the matrix to the outer membrane space. Why? Because remember that $FADH_2$ enters at complex II, rather than complex I, resulting in less overall energy captured, and fewer protons pumped from the matrix to the outer membrane space (see Figure 2.9). For three protons pumped, approximately one ATP can be generated. Thus, from NADH we can generate 10 protons, and 3.33 ATP molecules, while $FADH_2$ would generate 6 protons, and thus 2.0

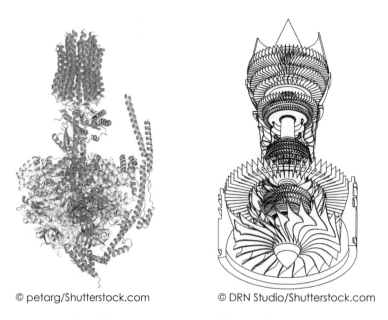

© petarg/Shutterstock.com   © DRN Studio/Shutterstock.com

Figure 2.10: **ATP Synthase.** The ATP Synthase enzymes looks like a jet engine turbine, and similarly, gives power to the cell, in the form of ATP

ATP molecules. BUT, didn't we say earlier that there were only 2.5 ATP and 1.5 ATP per NADH and $FADH_2$ respectively? Why is it less than expected? Let's think about that...

Generally, energy is needed for transport of molecules into the mitochondria, and transport of ATP out of the mitochondria. For example, protons are transported across the mitochondrial membrane as a consequence of the transport of ADP, ATP, and inorganic phosphate (P_i) in and out of the mitochondria. Based on these factors, we can safely assume that we get a *net gain* of one ATP from every 4 protons—thus for the 10 protons pumped for 1 NADH and the 6 protons pumped for 1 $FADH_2$, 4 ATP total can be made (2.5 and 1.5, respectively).

To summarize, the coordinated activity of the TCA and ETC cycles constitute the oxidative phosphorylation process. This process starts with acetyl CoA that is produced from the oxidation of macronutrients (carbohydrates, fats, and proteins) that moves into the TCA cycle, generating NADH and $FADH_2$ for proton pumping through the ETC, and eventual generation of ATP.

Reactive Oxygen Species and Oxidative Stress

The generation of ATP from mitochondria is not without some byproducts. Water is one of these (Complex IV). The other byproducts that are produced are reactive oxygen species or "ROS". In fact, ~99+% of all ROS in the cell comes from the mitochondria doing its "normal business"—making energy. Production of ROS is a normal process, and in fact, in some cells, ROS is harvested for cellular processes (i.e. immune cells kill bacteria with them). ROS levels also signal that there is a "stressor" going on, and that the cell needs to respond to these.

So, what are these ROS molecules and how are they made? ROS are generated when there is incomplete oxidation of oxygen—termed superoxide that happens when one molecule of oxygen, which normally should accept 4 protons to make water (H_2O), doesn't, becoming incompletely oxidized, or as shown, an oxygen radical:

$$O_2 + 1\ e^- \rightarrow O_2^- \text{ (superoxide anion)}$$

The superoxide anions can be made at several steps in the ETC—specifically in those steps where there is proton pumping (complex I, III, and IV—most documented in complexes I and III[13]) (Figure 2.9). It is estimated that $0.2 - 2.0\%$ of all oxygen taken into the mitochondria, results in superoxide formation[13]. So every place where you see proton generation, you will have ROS production.

Why? It turns out that there is a higher percentage of oxygen being reduced, or not completely oxidized to H_2O when an individual is at rest and when ATP demands are being met. When there is low ETC flux or activity, such as when ADP levels are low, and ATP levels are high, there is likely to also be a higher NADH supply than is needed, and thus higher delivery of electrons to the ETC than is needed, along with ample oxygen. This causes electrons to leak resulting in superoxide anion formation. The lipid coenzyme Q, which shuttles electrons from both complex I and complex II to complex III, can be present in three forms—CoQ ubiquione (oxidized), CoQ ubisemiquinone (partially reduced) and $CoQH_2$ ubiquinol (fully reduced) (Figure 2.11). The longer that the partially reduced ubisemiquinone form hangs around, the more likely that it will donate electrons, forming superoxide anions.

How do we combat this? We don't want oxygen radicals hanging around for too long. Almost an immediate response to the generation of oxygen radicals, a process called "uncoupling" is

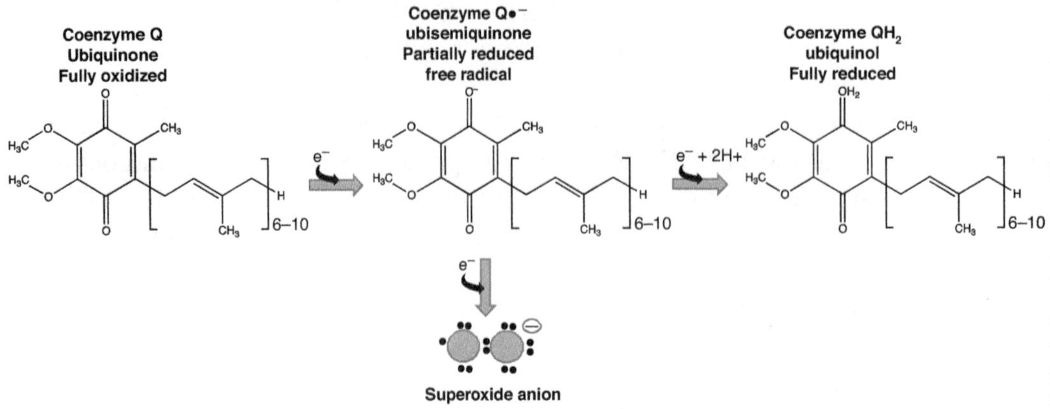

Figure 2.11: **States of Co-enzyme Q.** Coenzyme Q can exist in three oxidation states, depending on electron availability. Ubisemiquinone can donate electrons and form superoxide anions.

unleashed. Essentially a "hole" is poked in the inner membrane by inserting an uncoupling protein, and this effectively reduces the proton motive force (i.e. number of protons in the inner membrane space). Most mitochondria are "somewhat" uncoupled...in other words, we lose protons by having them leak out of the inner membrane space into the matrix, so that these protons are never coupled to make ATP by ATP synthase. Heat is the byproduct.

Heat—that's interesting right? Yes, uncoupling proteins allow protons to return to the matrix side of the mitochondrial membrane, and in brown adipose tissue this is a really important process because the heat

> **Big thoughts...**
>
> Brown adipose tissue (BAT) in humans is sparse, when compared to other animals. Many grants at the National Institutes of Health are focused on trying to identify mechanisms (Drugs? Foods? Exercises?) that might increase human BAT levels. Why? If you guessed to promote reduced body weight you guessed correctly...but will that work?

generated helps with thermogenesis in infants. Thus, we can generate body heat through this uncoupling process, that occurs in most of our body's mitochondria, but predominately in brown adipose tissue. Transcription of uncoupling proteins (UCPs) is increased in response to superoxide production, in a fasting state, or with long term calorie restriction—notice that all of these, are situations where the ATP/ADP ratios may favor a lower level of ADP and higher level of ATP. Alternatively, transcription of UCPs tend to decrease with exercise. There, the ATP needs are great, and ATP levels are likely lower than ADP levels. It all makes sense right?

There are three UCP isoforms, and each of these isoforms are tissue specific and has its own role. UCP1 is predominately found in brown fat, where, as mentioned above, the uncoupling process is mainly linked to the generation of heat (for a recent review see[14]). There are lots of brown fat depots in rodents and in infant humans. In rodents, these brown adipose tissue (BAT) pads are found around the scapula, while in humans, the BAT is more diffuse, and not found in pads, but it is found within other fat depots, as well as in muscle, and skin. For the other two uncoupling protein isoforms, UCP2 is a more universal uncoupling protein, found in many different tissues, while UCP3 is predominately a muscle-specific protein where the energy needs of the muscles are finely tuned to energy needs, by dumping the excess protons when needs are low[15].

Balancing Production and Neutralization of Free Radicals

The production of free radicals can't go on untethered without systems in place to neutralize them. Of course, our body and its individual cells have developed processes to neutralize the free radicals generated by the ETC. There are both enzymatic antioxidants, and non-enzymatic antioxidants that work in concert in all body systems to prevent the balance from tipping and allowing too many free radicals to be roaming around and attacking our cells, and the proteins, fats, and nucleic acids in them. These systems can adapt—in other words, when there is increased production of superoxide and hydrogen peroxide, this can be sensed, and neutralized quickly. So how is this done?

Superoxide

Superoxide, which we previously saw produced in the ETC, has several routes for neutralization. First, it can migrate away from the mitochondria. This is less likely, as usually hydrogen peroxide migrates out of the mitochondria, but not superoxide. Within the mitochondria, superoxide can dismutate to hydrogen peroxide. This is also not a common route, because the reaction is quite slow. The primary fate for superoxide is enzymatic dismutation—or dismutation by a class of enzymes that convert superoxide to hydrogen peroxide. These enzymes, called "superoxide dismutases" or SODs use the following enzymatic reaction:

$$2\ O_2^- + 2H^+ \rightarrow H_2O_2 + O_2$$

There are two main SODs—MnSOD and Cu/ZnSOD, named such by the metal ion that sits at their core (Figure 2.12). MnSOD has a manganese ion and is also called SOD2. This SOD sits within the mitochondria, and is a primary route by which mitochondrial-generated superoxide is neutralized to hydrogen peroxide. Cu/ZnSOD,

Did you know...?

Manganese, copper and zinc are micronutrients that are needed in specific quantities by the body—at least in part because of their roles in neutralizing free radicals.

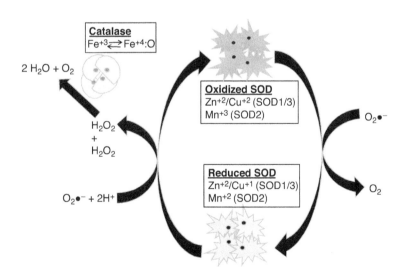

Figure 2.12: Mammalian Superoxide Dismutases (SODs). SODs are composed of either two (SOD1) or four (SOD2, and SOD3) identical subunits (blue), each with a mineral-containing active site (either copper/zinc or manganese, black dot). Catalase can take care of excess H_2O_2 produced during the reaction, and requires the mineral iron to do so.

which is also called SOD1, has both a zinc and a copper ion at its core, with zinc not being needed for the reaction but provides higher thermal stability[16]. This enzyme is found in the cytoplasm, acting as a defense against any superoxide that migrates into the cytoplasm, or is generated in other enzymatic processes.

Hydrogen Peroxide

We've seen above that SODs, as well as the other processes, generate hydrogen peroxide from superoxide. But hydrogen peroxide isn't exactly a great thing to hang around in our cells, as it is also an oxidizer. In the body, spontaneous decomposition occurs, but luckily, there are several systems that work to take care of hydrogen peroxides that are generated—catalase, the glutathione system, peroxiredoxins, and thioredoxoins. Let's take a look at each of these.

Catalase is a fantastic enzyme for a cell to have, and because of that, all living organisms that are exposed to oxygen have a catalase enzyme to deal with hydrogen peroxide. Catalase can convert hydrogen peroxide (H_2O_2) to water—with just one catalase enzyme capable of converting millions of H_2O_2 molecules to water and oxygen in a *single second* (Figure 2.12). Now that's a hard-working enzyme!

> **Did you know...?**
> Hydrogen peroxide lying around your bathroom cabinet, the longer it is exposed to air and light, the more likely that you don't have as strong of a solution as you did when you first bought it. That's why hydrogen peroxide is usually sold in brown, light-proof bottles. Keep the cap tight, and the bottle at normal room temperature, and you should have a good disinfectant for at least a couple of years..

The glutathione system utilizes reduced glutathione molecules to reduce H_2O_2 molecules to water and oxygen as well, via the enzyme glutathione peroxidase (Figure 2.13). With this system, oxidized glutathione is produced, but the enzyme glutathione reductase with one NADPH can regenerate the glutathione so that it is ready to tackle more H_2O_2. Of note, NADPH can be produced by the pentose phosphate pathway, and we will talk more about that pathway in glucose catabolism in the chapter 7.

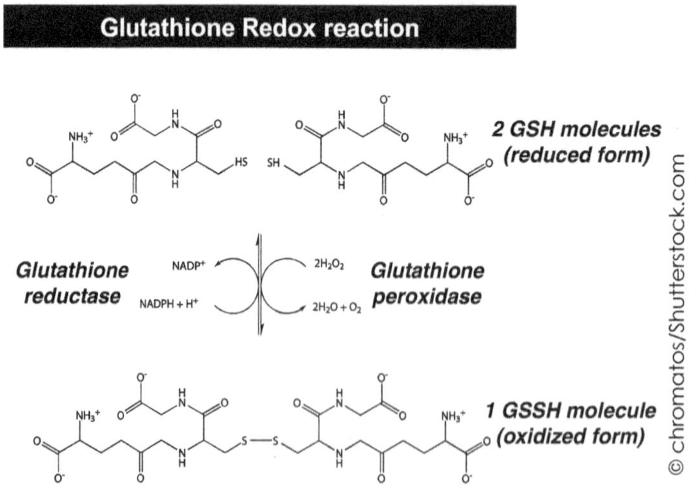

Glutathione Redox reaction

2 GSH molecules (reduced form)

Glutathione reductase — $NADP^+$, $NADPH + H^+$

Glutathione peroxidase — $2H_2O_2$, $2H_2O + O_2$

1 GSSH molecule (oxidized form)

© chromatos/Shutterstock.com

Figure 2.13: **The Glutathione System.** Hydrogen peroxide is reduced using 2 glutathione molecules and the enzyme glutathione peroxidase, producing one oxidized molecule of glutathione (GSSH). This can be reduced by the glutathione reductase enzyme, but requires utilizing an NADPH plus a proton.

Peroxiredoxins and thioredoxins are cysteine-based peroxidases that recently have been found to not only be involved in H_2O_2 dissipation, but also in cellular signaling[17]. While that latter function is beyond the scope of this chapter, it is important to realize that the peroxiredoxins and thioredoxins use the sulfur molecules of cysteine amino acids contained in their structure, to capture and then neutralize reactive oxygens, resulting in the production of water molecules. These thiol groups are oxidized from $[SH_2—SH_2]$ to $[S—S]$ during the process. There are two thioredoxin proteins in humans, thioredoxin (TXN) and thioredoxin-2 (TXN2), which do not directly reduce H_2O_2, but rather act to regenerate (reduce) other proteins, such as oxidized peroxiredoxin mentioned below. Both TXN and TXN2 are regenerated back to their reduced state using the enzyme thioredoxin reductase in an NADPH-dependent reaction. Note again the use of NADPH for this reaction. The peroxiredoxins are a family of six enzymes in humans, and these enzymes can regenerate or neutralize H_2O_2 to 2 water molecules. The oxidized peroxiredoxins then use reduced thioredoxin to regenerate and become ready to attack more H_2O_2 molecules.

Summary

Energy generation is necessary to life, and our individual cells have evolved systems to create ATP from macronutrient energy sources. However, as we've seen, energy generation has some costs, including the generation of free radicals and superoxide molecules. Cells have also evolved mechanisms to deal with these or even use them in cellular defense. The end result is that water, oxygen, and ATP are produced and can be used by the cell for other reactions.

Points to Ponder

➤ What would happen to an organism that couldn't make uncoupling proteins? Can you find an example of this in the literature?

➤ What do you think of the theory that electron transport chain complexes are composed of both mitochondrial and nuclear genes due to a symbiotic relationship that developed between an early (say millions of years ago) cell, and a bacterial-like organism? Look up the term symbiogenesis for more information.

➤ How are superoxides or other free radicals captured and used by immune cells?

References

1. Guimaraes-Ferreira L. Role of the phosphocreatine system on energetic homeostasis in skeletal and cardiac muscles. *Einstein (Sao Paulo)*. 2014;12(1):126–131.
2. Rampelt H, van der Laan M. Metabolic remodeling: a pyruvate transport affair. *EMBO J.* 2015; 34(7):835–837.
3. Lanhers C, Pereira B, Naughton G, Trousselard M, Lesage FX, Dutheil F. Creatine Supplementation and Upper Limb Strength Performance: A Systematic Review and Meta-Analysis. *Sports Med.* 2017;47(1):163–173.
4. Lanhers C, Pereira B, Naughton G, Trousselard M, Lesage FX, Dutheil F. Creatine Supplementation and Lower Limb Strength Performance: A Systematic Review and Meta-Analyses. *Sports Med.* 2015;45(9):1285–1294.
5. Butts J, Jacobs B, Silvis M. Creatine Use in Sports. *Sports Health*. 2018;10(1):31–34.

6. Atlante A, Seccia TM, Marra E, Passarella S. The rate of ATP export in the extramitochondrial phase via the adenine nucleotide translocator changes in aging in mitochondria isolated from heart left ventricle of either normotensive or spontaneously hypertensive rats. *Mech Ageing Dev.* 2011;132(10):488–495.

7. Maldonado EN, DeHart DN, Patnaik J, Klatt SC, Gooz MB, Lemasters JJ. ATP/ADP Turnover and Import of Glycolytic ATP into Mitochondria in Cancer Cells Is Independent of the Adenine Nucleotide Translocator. *J Biol Chem.* 2016;291(37):19642–19650.

8. The Nobel Prize in Physiology or Medicine 1953 1953; http://www.nobelprize.org/nobel_prizes/medicine/laureates/1953/>. Accessed 21 February, 2018.

9. Duckworth HW, Nguyen NT, Gao Y, et al. Enzyme-substrate complexes of allosteric citrate synthase: evidence for a novel intermediate in substrate binding. *Biochim Biophys Acta.* 2013;1834(12):2546–2553.

10. Treves C, Vincenzini MT, Vanni P, Iantomasi T, Stio M, Baccari V. Activities of NAD-and NADP-specific isocitrate dehydrogenases in kidney mitochondria of rachitic rat. *Biochem Cell Biol.* 1986;64(12):1310–1316.

11. Denton RM. Regulation of mitochondrial dehydrogenases by calcium ions. *Biochim Biophys Acta.* 2009;1787(11):1309–1316.

12. "Peter Mitchell - Facts". 1978; https://www.nobelprize.org/nobel_prizes/chemistry/laureates/1978/mitchell-facts.html. Accessed Feb 14, 2018.

13. Li X, Fang P, Mai J, Choi ET, Wang H, Yang XF. Targeting mitochondrial reactive oxygen species as novel therapy for inflammatory diseases and cancers. *J Hematol Oncol.* 2013;6:19.

14. Chouchani ET, Kazak L, Spiegelman BM. Mitochondrial reactive oxygen species and adipose tissue thermogenesis: Bridging physiology and mechanisms. *J Biol Chem.* 2017;292(41):16810–16816.

15. Bouillaud F, Alves-Guerra MC, Ricquier D. UCPs, at the interface between bioenergetics and metabolism. *Biochim Biophys Acta.* 2016;1863(10):2443–2456.

16. Culotta VC, Yang M, O'Halloran TV. Activation of superoxide dismutases: putting the metal to the pedal. *Biochim Biophys Acta.* 2006;1763(7):747–758.

17. Netto LE, Antunes F. The Roles of Peroxiredoxin and Thioredoxin in Hydrogen Peroxide Sensing and in Signal Transduction. *Mol Cells.* 2016;39(1):65–71.

CHAPTER 3

Macronutrient Metabolism: Turning Carbohydrates into Usable Energy

The food we eat becomes the energy that we need to run enzymatic processes in our bodies. As we will see in the next three chapters, the processes for turning carbohydrates, lipids (fats), and proteins into usable energy (ATP) are slightly different, but still converge on the TCA and ETC pathways discussed in Chapter 2. In this chapter, we will focus on carbohydrates as a starting point, and also discuss how we store usable energy that is derived from carbohydrates.

Carbohydrate Metabolism

The body goes to extreme measures to make sure that carbohydrate metabolism is controlled at many levels. Let's talk about metabolism and think about why control of carbohydrate metabolism is so important.

Carbohydrates come in two main flavors—namely simple carbohydrates and complex carbohydrates (Figure 3.1). However, for both of these forms, glucose is the main end product that the body produces and regulates. Simple carbohydrates can be further subdivided into mono- and disaccharides. While monosaccharides (glucose, fructose, and galactose) can be directly absorbed and used, disaccharides (lactose, sucrose, and maltose) are further broken down in the small intestine to their monosaccharide components. Complex carbohydrates also have two main forms—oligo- and polysaccharides. While the oligosaccharides have 3-10 simple carbohydrates, polysaccharides have more

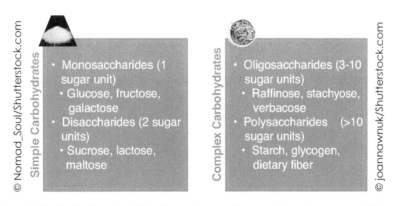

Figure 3.1: **Categories of Carbohydrates.** Simple and complex carbohydrates are delineated by the number of sugar units present in the molecule. Most complex carbohydrates can be broken down further into monosaccharide units.

than 10, and include the more difficult to digest starch—dietary fiber. Starch, which can range in size from a few thousand to 500,000 units, can be broken down into glucose in the small intestine, which again can be directly used for energy-generating pathways. On the other hand, we cannot break down dietary fiber, but bacteria in our guts can do that. Of course, the result is usually gas (in the form of methane) and short chain fatty acids.

Not all carbohydrates are created equally. And what we mean by this is that not all are linear units of saccharides strung together in a chain. For starch, there are two main types that we find in edible plants—amylose and amylopectin. While amylose is linear, amylopectin is highly branched. Glycogen, which serves as the main storage unit for glucose in animals is also highly branched, in fact it is about two times more branched than amylopectin. This branching allows for glucoses to be "pulled off" enzymatically more readily because there are more sites per molecule for enzymes to act on, when glucose is in demand. Glycogen is stored in the liver and in muscle. Liver glycogen is the main source of glucose that is used to maintain blood glucose levels. Glycogen stored in muscle is a very important local source of glucose for muscle in times of rapid energy demand, during exercise for example. While muscle can store large amounts of glycogen and hydrolyze it quickly when needed, it cannot release glucose, from hydrolyzed glycogen, into the blood like the liver does. When muscle glycogen is broken down, glucose-6-phosphate is produced, and this directly feeds into glycolysis for either aerobic or anaerobic metabolism, and ATP production.

> **Did you know...?**
>
> Prebiotics, which are sold over the counter are usually made up of oligosaccharides, and if the right combination is picked, these can promote the growth of "good" bacteria (*Bifidobacteria and Lactobacillus*) in our guts.

Keeping Blood Glucose Levels in Check

As mentioned previously in this section, the body goes to extremes to keep blood glucose levels in check. Let's talk about that—specifically what, how, when, and where. As shown on Table 3.1, the normal fasting blood glucose range (clinically measured in mg of glucose per deciliter of blood, or mg/dl) is in the range of 90-126. So, if you go into the physician and have a casual blood glucose level of 110 mg/dl, then all is well. However, if your value were to read >126 or <54, then you would be considered hyper- or hypoglycemic, respectively.

> **The LIVER-a major organ for glucose homeostasis**
>
> While we usually think of the liver as the place where toxins are neutralized, the liver is also the main way in which blood glucose levels can be modulated in response to changing needs. It does this by using its glycogen stores as a source of glucose molecules for secretion.

Why is this important? As shown on Figure 3.2, normal glucose output from the liver is approximately 150 mg/min, while normal glucose usage by red blood cells, the brain, and all of the other cells in your body is also approximately 150 mg/min. These amounts are the same right? However, if you start exercising, glucose needs might go up to 950 mg/min, especially because the muscles have much greater need for glucose during exercise. In a normal, healthy person, the liver will respond to this need by secreting about 5-8 times more glucose. This takes care of the extra need by the muscles, and still leaves enough to supply tissues such as red blood cells, the brain, and the renal medulla—tissues that can *only* use glucose as a fuel source. In

Table 3.1   **Categories of Glycemia.**

	Glucose concentration	
	(mM)	(mg/dL)
Euglycemia[a] (normal range)	5-7	90-126
Hypoglycemia[b] (low blood glucose)	<3	< 54
Hyperglycemia[c] (high blood glucose)	>7	>126

[a]Normal blood glucose levels will range, depending on time after a meal or during exercise. [b]Arbitrary definition as people may exhibit symptoms at higher values than this. Low values obtained with fasting or prolonged exercise. [c]High blood sugar, especially when an individual has been fasting is indicative of diabetes.

addition, the small intestine will ramp up transport of glucose into your bloodstream, if you are within about 1-6 hours of your last meal, depending on the carbohydrate content of that meal. Generally, after we eat a meal, glucose levels rise (as does insulin- more on that later), due to food-based glucose absorption.

Of note, while Figure 3.2 shows the liver ramping up glucose secretion, it turns out that in addition to the liver, there is a small contribution from the kidneys[1], and astrocytes in the brain[2], as

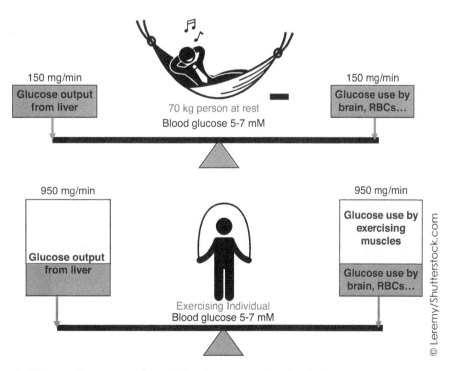

Figure 3.2: **Blood Glucose Homeostasis.** While glucose needs of individual tissues are different at rest or while exercising, in normal healthy individuals, blood glucose levels stay within a very tight range.

kidneys and astrocytes of the brain can also use the process of gluconeogenesis to make glucose from non-carbohydrate sources. These non-carbohydrate sources include lactate, glycerol, and the carbon backbones of amino acids.

Removing Glucose from the Blood- Harder than adding it!

If there is too much glucose in the blood, our systems try to get levels back into that normal range of 90-126 mg/dl by having cells that might use it,

> **The low carb diet**
>
> What happens when you go on a low carb diet? How does this affect glycogen stores? Consider how a low carb diet might affect the balance of gluconeogenesis to glycolysis in your body.

transport the glucose out of the blood and into the cells. These cells, such as muscle cells and liver cells, will respond by either using the glucose (when energy needs are high) or storing it as glycogen or as lipids (if carbohydrate intake is too high compared to energy demand-more about this later in the book). In the muscle, whether or not the glucose is used or stored depends on when you've had your last meal, and whether you are using your muscles—ultimately the state of "energy balance" in your body at that time. It also depends on the type of muscle fiber we are talking about. Adipose tissue uses what glucose it needs, and then predominately stores the rest as fat, while liver, again will use some, but then store the rest as glycogen, with a little bit as fat. Have you ever heard of fatty liver? This sometimes occurs in obese individuals[3] (Figure 3.3), and likely is due to the liver taking more glucose than is needed for glycogen storage, which then can be used for *de novo* fat synthesis, specifically making new fatty acids and storing them as triglycerides. Excess fructose consumption in the diet can also contribute to increased *de novo* fat synthesis in the liver. On the other hand, most other tissues use glucose for energy and don't really uptake glucose unless these need it. The brain is a great example of this—and is a major user of glucose. Think about lightheadedness that occurs when you stand up, especially if you haven't eaten in a while…this in part is due to

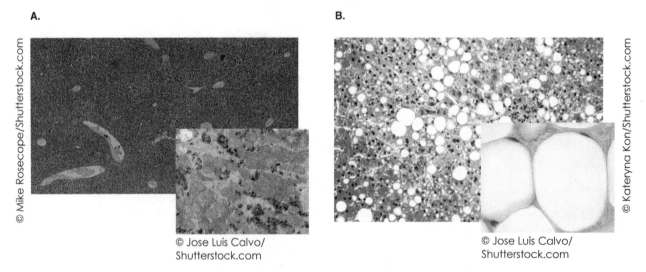

A.   © Mike Rosecope/Shutterstock.com

© Jose Luis Calvo/
Shutterstock.com

B.   © Kateryna Kon/Shutterstock.com

© Jose Luis Calvo/
Shutterstock.com

Figure 3.3: **Liver.** A normal, healthy liver, contains about 7% of its weight in glycogen (**A**). Inset shows a digitally-enhanced transmission electron microscope view of a single liver cell where the mitochondria are blue, the endoplasmic reticulum are brown, and the glycogen is pink. (**B**) A fatty liver still contains glycogen but also lots of adipose (fat) cells. The inset shown the fat cells, with large intercellular lipids, and the nucleus flattened and to the edge of the cell.

lower than normal blood glucose levels[4] (along with a drop in blood pressure upon standing). Of note, astrocytes (which are a type of neuroglial cell and not neurons), can both synthesize glycogen, and break down glycogen to deliver glucose to neurons[5].

Glycogen is the ultimate storage molecule for glucose. It is the carbohydrate composition of the diet and the body's needs that determine how much total glycogen is stored. Glycogen is a very compact structure that allows for a lot of glucose to be stored in a very small amount of space. The liver stores large amounts of glycogen. As a whole, this means that about 7% of the entire wet weight of a fresh liver is made up of glycogen (Figure 3.3). Muscle on the other hand has about 1% of its mass as glycogen, which is less per unit of the organ, when compared to liver, but because muscle tissue makes up so much more of the body than liver tissue (i.e. 32kg of a normal 70kg man, and 22 kg of a normal 55 kg woman, as compared to 1.2kg and 1.0kg of liver, respectively), we actually store much more *total* glycogen in the muscle. And the muscle predominately uses its own glycogen stores to funnel glucose into glycolysis for ATP production.

Making and Breaking Sugars for Energy

Glycogenolysis

To maintain blood glucose levels or to have glucose available to produce ATP, we must release that glucose that has been stored as glycogen. Glycogenolysis is the process by which glycogen is broken down into individual glucose units that can feed into either glycolysis (in muscle) or into the blood stream for pick up by other tissues from the liver (Figure 3.4). In this process, the glycogen phosphorylase enzyme attacks a terminal alpha (α) 1-4 bond of glycogen and adds an inorganic phosphate to the glucose that is removed. Why doesn't this process use ATP like a lot of enzymes attaching phosphate molecules? Because the breaking of the (α) 1-4 bond releases enough energy alone for the reaction to proceed[6]. The glycogen debranching enzyme (easy name to remember!) catalyzes a breaking of the (α) 1-6 branch points to release any other glucose molecules at

> **Genetic glycogen storage diseases**
>
> There are many different forms of glycogen storage diseases, usually caused by mutations in one of the glycogen synthesis or glycogenolysis enzymes. For example, in glycogen storage disease I, there is an inactivating mutation in phosphoglucomutase. Babies have cleft lip, while adults show exercise intolerance. Check out other glycogen storage diseases using the Online Mendelian Inheritance in Man database (www.OMIM.org).

the branch point[7]. Glucose cannot immediately go in to glycolysis at this point as it is in the form glucose-1-phosphate. This molecule must be "transmutated" or, in other words, have its phosphate transferred, using the enzyme phosphoglucomutase from the number 1 carbon to the number 6 carbon. Now the glucose-6-phosphate molecule can be shuttled into glycolysis in muscle. In the liver there is another enzyme, glucose-6-phosphatase, whose role is to remove the phosphate from glucose-6-phosphate, allowing for glucose to be secreted into the blood.

As mentioned earlier, we must maintain blood glucose in a normal range. One way to do this is to keep adequate stores of glycogen. In glycogen synthesis (or glycogenesis), the glucose enters the liver cell (hepatocyte) or muscle cell and is converted to glucose-6-phosphate by hexokinase in muscle or glucokinase in liver. From there, glucose-6-phosphate can be converted to glucose-1-phosphate using the same enzyme that switched it in the first place—phosphoglucomutase. It then is conjugated to UDP, using the enzyme UDP-pyrophosphorylase, with UTP (uridine triphosphate) as a co-substrate in the reaction. Glycogen synthase can take the UDP-glucose and add it onto glycogen, using an (α) 1-4 bond, releasing the UDP. Finally, a glycogen branching

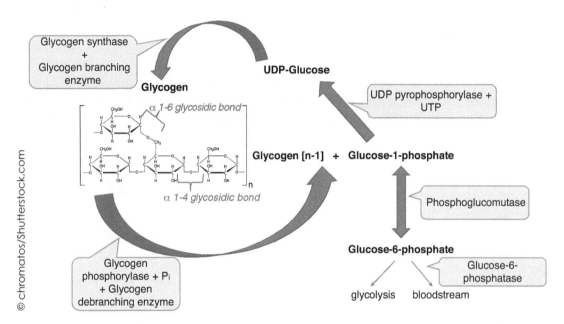

Figure 3.4: Glycogenolysis and Glycogen synthesis. Glycogenolysis is the breakdown of glycogen by debranching enzyme, and glycogen phosphorylase (plus inorganic phosphate), while glycogen synthesis takes one UDP-glucose and branching enzyme, which yields a longer glycogen molecule for storage. The glucose-1-phosphate produced from glycogenolysis cannot be used directly in glycolysis, but rather needs to be changed into glucose-6-phosphate using the enzyme phosphoglucomutase.

enzyme can form branch points in the glycogen molecule by introducing (α) 1-6 bonds at regular intervals[7]. Together, the breakdown and synthesis of glycogen gives our bodies the ability to either store, use, or transport glucose.

Glycolysis

In a fed state, when circulating glucose is high in the blood, glucose is the primary substrate for ATP production. We metabolize glucose (and fructose and galactose to a smaller extent), under both aerobic and anaerobic conditions, in glycolysis. Glycolysis has a few more steps than glycogenolysis. The process requires the investment of 2 ATP, but results in the production of 4 ATP and 2 NADH, meaning that there is a net energy gain. Sometimes you have to spend a little to make more—in business and in physiology. However, this is again different from glycogenolysis and glycogen synthesis, as there is no energy gains or losses during those processes.

The process of glycolysis is usually described as having three stages—the priming stage, the splitting stage, and the reducing/oxidizing stage (Figure 3.5). In the priming stage, glucose is phosphorylated by hexokinase (in muscle) or glucokinase (in liver) and this uses a phosphate from ATP, creating glucose-6-phosphate (G6P). As we saw above, G6P can also be derived directly from glycogen, and so glycolysis and glycogenolysis can work together to make ATP. If you look at the reaction, when G6P comes from glycogen, you don't have to use that extra ATP to convert it from glucose to G6P (producing a net of 3 ATP), compared to when a cell is using glucose directly from blood (producing a net of 2 ATP). G6P is then enzymatically converted to fructose-6-phosphate by the enzyme phosphohexose isomerase. This enzyme goes by several different names, including glucose-6-isomerase, and phosphoglucose isomerase, so don't be fooled by the nicknames. Next comes phosphofructose kinase I (PFK-1), which phosphorylates fructose-6-phosphate, forming fructose 1,6 bisphosphate. This reaction also requires ATP both for the transfer of the P_i moiety, as well as

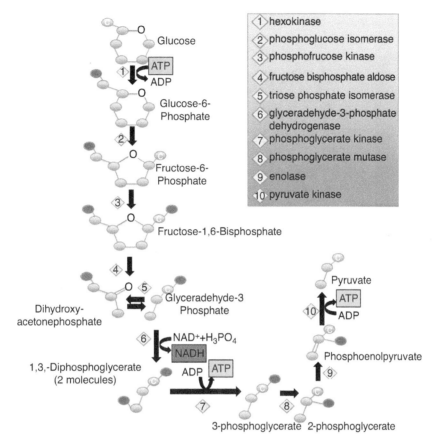

Figure 3.5: Glycolysis. The steps of glycolysis and enzymes catalyzing these steps are shown. ATP generation (green), and NADH generation (purple) are also shown.

energy for the reaction. The hexokinase and PFK-1 steps are rate-limiting steps in glycolysis. What this means is that at these points, glycolysis can be sped up or slowed down based on the activity of these enzymes. Hexokinase, because the phosphorylation of glucose traps it in the cell. The PFK-1 step is an important rate-limiting step because beyond this reaction, glucose is committed to glycolysis, whereas as prior to this step, G6P could be diverted to multiple other metabolic pathways, which include glycogen synthesis (discussed previously), or the pentose phosphate shuttle. In addition, fructose-6-phosphate, the product of phosphohexose isomerase, can be diverted into the hexosamine pathway. We will discuss these other pathways later, but because PFK-1 is the committed step to glycolysis and a primary control point, it also means that this point is highly regulated[8]. While we will talk about this extensively later, one example as to why PFK-1 is highly regulated has to do the energetic demands of the cell. PFK-1 is inhibited by high levels of ATP and stimulated by high levels of ADP. This makes sense because a cell would want to stimulate glycolysis if ATP levels are low and ADP levels are high, signaling that the cell needs to make more energy (ATP).

The splitting stage comes next, and this is where the fructose 1, 6 bisphosphate is cleaved into glyceraldehyde-3-phosphate and/or dihydroxyacetone phosphate. Dihydroxyacetone phosphate can either be converted into glyceraldehyde-3-phosphate via the action of triosephosphate isomerase or can be used for the synthesis of glycerol, the backbone of triglycerides. Of note, triosephosphate isomerase deficiency, which prevents the conversion of dihydroxyacetone phosphate to glyceraldehyde phosphate is the *only* glycolytic enzyme deficiency which is lethal in humans[9], lending credence to its importance in the conversion reaction.

The redox stage of glycolysis finishes everything up and creates metabolic energy for use down the line. The first step starts this energy production process off, with glyceraldehyde-3-phosphate dehydrogenase generating 2 NADH molecules and cleaving glyceraldehyde-3-phosphate to 1,3 bis-phosphoglycerate. This is the only step in glycolysis where NADH is formed, incidentally. The NADH has multiple fates, one of which is transferring electrons (protons) to the mitochondria via the glycerol-3-phosphate shuttle or the malate-aspartate shuttle for processing by the electron transport chain. Another possible fate of this NADH is that it could be oxidized in the lactate dehydrogenase reaction to make lactate from pyruvate, which will be discussed on more detail later. Four ATP molecules are made during the rest of glycolysis, specifically by the two kinase enzymes—phosphoglycerate kinase and pyruvate kinase, providing a net production of two ATP. From there, pyruvate is the end product of glycolysis, but not the end of energy production!

Pyruvate

While pyruvate is the end product of glycolysis, from there it has two fates—the pyruvate can either be directly shuttled into the mitochondria or it can be reduced to lactate using the enzyme lactate dehydrogenase. In an anaerobic state when the latter reaction is used, then NADH, which was generated during glycolysis, is oxidized back to NAD^+ by the lactate dehydrogenase enzyme. As this reaction takes place in the cytoplasm, the NADH generated during glycolysis is used and maintains the NAD^+ pool for glycolysis to continue. However, in an aerobic state we go a different route, and pyruvate enters the mitochondria. The NADH from the splitting stage needs to be shuttled into the mitochondria, as NADH is impermeable to the mitochondrial membrane. Let's talk about how this works.

Electrons from NADH are shuttled into the mitochondria using the glycerol-3-phosphate shuttle or the malate aspartate shuttle (Figure 3.6 and 3.7). In the glycerol-3-phosphate shuttle process, NADH transfers its electrons to a glycolysis intermediate, dihydroxyacetone phosphate (DHAP) producing glycerol-3-phosphate (G3P), via the glycerol 3-phosphate dehydrogenase enzyme. G3P can shuttle through the outer mitochondrial membrane, and as the mitochondrial glycerol 3-phosphate dehydrogenase enzyme sits on the inner mitochondrial membrane, the G3P electrons are transferred to the FAD in Complex II of the electron transport chain, making $FADH_2$ and DHAP. The electrons from $FADH_2$ are then transferred to co-enzyme Q of the ETC. Note that DHAP can be shuttled back out of the mitochondria for use again by the cytoplasmic glycerol-3-phosphate dehydrogenase. Therefore, there is no net consumption of substrates or products, just the transferring of electrons. The glycerol-3 phosphate shuttle is actually the less prominent shuttle to transfer NADH electrons into the mitochondrial membrane for most cell types. However, in fast glycolytic skeletal muscle fibers, this is the predominant NADH shuttle system, and expression of the mitochondrial glycerol-3-phosphate enzyme itself is high in brown adipose tissue, brain, and skeletal muscle[10]. A total of 3 ATPs can ultimately be generated from the electron transport chain and ATP synthase using this shuttle system to transfer the 2 NADH derived from one glucose molecule in glycolysis.

Most other tissues use the more common malate-aspartate shuttle (Figure 3.7). The same two NADH molecules from glycolysis can be processed into 5 ATP molecules by the electron transport chain and ATP synthase, making it a more energetically efficient method. To start this process, electrons from NADH are transferred to oxaloacetate forming malate, in the cytoplasm via malate dehydrogenase. Malate can take the extra electrons into the mitochondrial matrix, where malate is oxidized back to oxaloacetate by malate dehydrogenase and the electrons are transferred onto NAD^+, producing NADH within the mitochondria. The NADH can then be directly shuttled to complex I of the electron transport chain. Again, there is no net consumption of substrates or products, just the transferring of electrons.

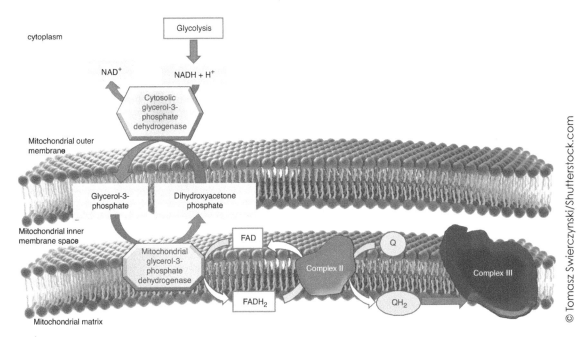

Figure 3.6: **The Glycerol-3-Phosphate Shuttle.** One of the fates of the NADH produced from glycolysis is use in the electron transport chain. However, NADH cannot cross the mitochondrial membrane, so the energy in NADH is transferred to glycerol-3-phosphate through cytosolic glycerol-3-phosphate dehydrogenase. Glycerol-3-phosphate can be shuttled into the inner membrane space of the mitochondria, where mitochondrial glycerol-3-phosphate dehydrogenase can transfer the electrons to FAD making $FADH_2$. This occurs at complex II in the electron transport system, where the electrons from $FADH_2$ can then be transferred to co-enzyme Q, forming QH_2 which can enter complex III. A total of 3 ATP can be generated from the initial 2 NADH made from glycolysis this way.

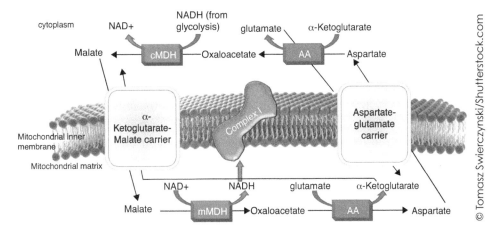

Figure 3.7: **The Malate-Aspartate Shuttle.** NADH produced from glycolysis can also use the Malate-Aspartate Shuttle to be used in the electron transport chain. Again, NADH cannot cross the mitochondrial membrane, so with this shuttle system, the energy in NADH is transferred to oxalacetate using the cytoplasmic enzyme malate dehydrogenase (cMDH). Malate then uses the α ketoglutarate-malate carrier to transfer malate into the mitochondrial matrix. The reverse set of reactions now take place, converting the energy in malate to oxaloacetate, using the mitochondrial form of MDH (mMDH) and forming NADH from NAD^+. The NADH can be directly used by Complex I of the electron transport chain, generating a total of 5 ATPs from the initial 2 NADH from glycolysis. Aspartate aminotransferase enzyme (AA) is needed to complete the reaction process. The aspartate from the end reaction is transported back out to the cytoplasm for re-use in the Malate-Aspartate Shuttle.

So what about the other pyruvate fate–the one involving lactate production? Any time glycolysis occurs (i.e. when we have glucose coming into the cell), lactate can be produced. However, the rate of lactate production will change based on glycolytic flux. What is meant by this is that during certain conditions such as physical activity, increased blood glucose levels (i.e. high carbohydrate meal), high muscle glycogen levels, when blood flow is reduced, or if the blood has a low oxygen content for other reasons lactate will be predominately produced. All of these conditions might contribute to a more anaerobic setting for the cell, (lack of O_2) and a reduced overall mitochondrial activity, or reduced oxidative capacity of the mitochondria, leading to the alternative pathway.

Sore muscles are not caused by lactic acid buildup!

While many of us have been told that lactate build-up in the muscles actually cause muscle soreness, this is NOT true. It is actually the microtears in muscle that occur concomitantly with strenuous physical activity (and lactate production) that cause the soreness. Pass that correct information on!

Muscle fiber types use lactate differently. In fact, the reaction shown below can go in either direction, but depending on the fiber type, one direction is favored over another. In slow oxidative fibers, or at times when we are in an aerobic state, the reaction tends to go in the direction of lactate oxidation, forming pyruvate and NADH. However, in fast glycolytic fibers, or during conditions of low oxygen, the reaction tends to go in the direction of pyruvate reduction, and the formation of lactate. However, while one might want to assume that lactate production is a *bad* thing, it isn't. Lactate has plenty of energy to give. This is a main concept in metabolic flexibility—in that multiple substrates can be used for energy production, and our bodies adapt to these different situations.

Lactate Dehydrogenase (LDH) enzyme catalyzes this reversible reaction shown below:

Pyruvate + NADH +H$^+$ ⟷ Lactate + NAD$^+$

Lactate dehydrogenase

There are multiple forms of LDH, all composed of one of three different subunits (Table 3.2). The predominant ones use the "heart" form of the protein (made from the LDHB gene) or the "muscle" form of the protein (from the LDHA gene). As each LDH enzyme is composed of four subunits, each isoform is one of five combinations of either the heart or muscle forms of LDH subunits. There is also a testis-specific form (from the LDHC gene), and that form is composed just of LDHC subunits[11]. The forward reaction is going to be favored when anaerobic conditions exist, but when aerobic conditions return, pyruvate and NADH can be made in the reverse reaction. Because pyruvate enters the mitochondria and is converted to acetyl CoA (and this can enter into the TCA cycle), up to 15 ATP molecules can be made from a single lactate molecule.

As we finish up glycolysis then, we need to step back and count our net energy production. First, in glycolysis there are the 2 ATP and the 2 NADH (3 or 5 ATP) molecules produced—but both of these are dependent on the glycerol-3-phosphate or the malate-aspartate shuttle systems to feed them into the ETC and produce ATP. There are also 2 NADH (5 ATP) molecules produced from pyruvate dehydrogenase conversion of 2 pyruvate to 2 acetyl-CoA. The 2 acetyl CoA molecules entering the TCA cycle go on to produce 6 NADH (15 ATP), 2 FADH$_2$ (3 ATP), and 2 GTP (2 ATP). Together these produce 30-32 ATP molecules per unit of glucose in aerobic metabolism.

Wait—why is there a range? We have differences in how NADH from glycolysis is shuttled into the mitochondria for use in electron transport. If we use the glycerol-3-phosphate shuttle, cytosolic NADH is transferred to make FADH$_2$ in the mitochondria producing the equivalent of 1.5 ATPs.

In the malate-aspartate shuttle, cytosolic NADH is transferred to make NADH in the mitochondria producing the equivalent of 2.5 ATP. Depending on which is used, this results in a net range of 30-32 total ATP molecules per unit of glucose used.

Table 3.2: **Lactase Dehydrogenase Enzyme.** The lactate dehydrogenase (LDH) enzyme comes in five different forms, formed by "heart" (H) and "muscle" (M) specific subunits in different combinations. The "H" and "M" subunits are derived from different genes, the LDHB, and LDHA genes respectively, making different proteins, which are then assembled into the different LDH forms. There is one unique LDH which is formed from the testis-specific LDH subunit gene, LDHC. This form appears to be only made in testes.

LDH Form	Subunit Composition		Distribution
LDH1	H4		Cardiac muscle Slow oxidative skeletal (Type I) muscle fibers
LDH2	M1, H3		Cardiac muscle Slow oxidative skeletal (Type I) muscle fibers
LDH3	M2, H2		Lung Kidney
LDH4	M3, H1		Kidney Fast glycolytic skeletal (Type II) muscle fibers
LDH5	M4		Liver Fast glycolytic skeletal (Type I) muscle fibers
LDH-C	T4		Testes

Summary

The body tightly controls how much circulating glucose is available—making sure there is enough, but not too much available for absorption by tissues. The brain, muscle, and liver are major players in glucose metabolism. From a starting point of one glucose molecule, our glucose molecule can have several different fates, and these different fates depend on whether there is a high or low energy demand and whether there is anaerobic or aerobic metabolism occurring. Make sure that you can calculate the different ATP amounts from the different fates for one glucose molecule.

Points to Ponder

➢ Physiologically, why is it so important to tightly control carbohydrates metabolism? Hint: think about what tissues rely primarily on carbohydrates.
➢ Is there a situation where a muscle might be taking in glucose and instead of using it, converting it to glycogen?

➣ When you break carbohydrate metabolism down to a basic unit, what substrates are we really interested in controlling?

➣ Why does the ATP generation from glycolysis derived NADH differ between the glycerol-3-phoshate vs. the malate-aspartate shuttle? Hint: think about NADH entering complex 1 of the ETC vs. $FADH_2$ entering the complex 2 of the ETC. Why does this matter?

References

1. Stumvoll M, Meyer C, Mitrakou A, Nadkarni V, Gerich JE. Renal glucose production and utilization: new aspects in humans. *Diabetologia.* 1997;40(7):749–757.

2. Yip J, Geng X, Shen J, Ding Y. Cerebral Gluconeogenesis and Diseases. *Front Pharmacol.* 2016;7:521.

3. Rinella ME. Nonalcoholic fatty liver disease: a systematic review. *JAMA.* 2015;313(22):2263–2273.

4. Wilson V. Non-diabetic hypoglycaemia: causes and pathophysiology. *Nurs Stand.* 2011;25(46):35–39.

5. Hertz L, Chen Y. Glycogenolysis, an Astrocyte-Specific Reaction, is Essential for Both Astrocytic and Neuronal Activities Involved in Learning. *Neuroscience.* 2018;370:27–36.

6. Bhagavan NV, Chung-Eun H. Carbohydrate Metabolism II: Gluconeogenesis, Glycogen Synthesis and Breakdown, and Alternative Pathways. In: *Essentials of Medical Biochemistry,* . San Diego: Academic Press; 2011:151–168.

7. Adeva-Andany MM, Gonzalez-Lucan M, Donapetry-Garcia C, Fernandez-Fernandez C, Ameneiros-Rodriguez E. Glycogen metabolism in humans. *BBA Clin.* 2016;5:85–100.

8. Mor I, Cheung EC, Vousden KH. Control of glycolysis through regulation of PFK1: old friends and recent additions. *Cold Spring Harb Symp Quant Biol.* 2011;76:211–216.

9. Orosz F, Olah J, Ovadi J. Triosephosphate isomerase deficiency: new insights into an enigmatic disease. *Biochim Biophys Acta.* 2009;1792(12):1168–1174.

10. Mracek T, Drahota Z, Houstek J. The function and the role of the mitochondrial glycerol-3-phosphate dehydrogenase in mammalian tissues. *Biochim Biophys Acta.* 2013;1827(3):401–410.

11. Storey KB. Comparative enzymology-new insights from studies of an "old" enzyme, lactate dehydrogenase. *Comp Biochem Physiol B Biochem Mol Biol.* 2016;199:13–20.

CHAPTER 4

Macronutrient Metabolism: Fats for Fuel

Lipids

As we move into lipid metabolism, we need to consider the various types of lipids that are *metabolizable*. Lipids are molecules that are soluble in non-polar substances—in other words, they are not soluble in water or in fluids that are charged. Lipids make up our cell membranes and travel through our blood as triglycerides from the gut in chylomicrons or from the liver as very-low density lipoproteins (VLDLs). As free fatty acids, lipids travel through the blood bound to albumin. For nutritional metabolism, we will consider only those lipids that we can metabolize—namely, the fatty acids, the glycerides, the non-glyceride lipids, and lipid carriers—lipoproteins (Figure 4.1).

Fatty acids come in two main flavors. Those with an even number of carbon atoms, which generally occur in nature, and those with an odd number of carbon atoms. The term "fatty acid" comes from the structure of the molecule, which has a carboxylic acid at one end, and a hydrocarbon chain extending from it. The hydrocarbon chains that occur in nature vary between 4 and 28 carbons[1], categorized as short (fewer than or equal to 5 carbons), medium (between 6 to 12 carbons), long (13 to 21 carbons, or very long (more than 22 carbons)[1].

Fatty acids can be further classified into saturated, and unsaturated, which describes the state of the carbon-carbon double bonds in the hydrocarbon tail (Figures 4.2 and 4.3). Saturated fatty acids have no carbon-carbon double bonds, while unsaturated fatty acids have at least one of these carbon-carbon double bonds. This might seem odd to you, but the saturation actually refers to whether all the carbons have the maximum amount of hydrogens attached. A saturated carbon-carbon bond has all hydrogens (2 on each carbon) associated with it, while an unsaturated carbon-carbon bond is double bonded and has only one hydrogen associated with it. Furthermore, a fatty acid that has only one of these double bonds is called a monounsaturated fatty acid or "MUFA", while a fatty acid containing two or more of these double bonds between carbons is called a polyunsaturated fatty acid or "PUFA". We can find saturated fatty acids predominately in coconut and palm oils, as well as meats, while unsaturated fatty acids are found in oils and nuts. When we think about a saturated fatty acid, consider that the structure of it allows for a more rigid form, as multiple fatty

> ### Fun Food Facts
> Hydrogenation was the food industry's way of making oils more stable (i.e. have a longer half-life). This process uses H_2 gas and nickel as a catalyst to create trans fats from unsaturated cis-fats. Trans fats generally do not occur in nature. Think of that next time you spread some margarine on your toast. The FDA is banning trans fats in foods as of 2018.

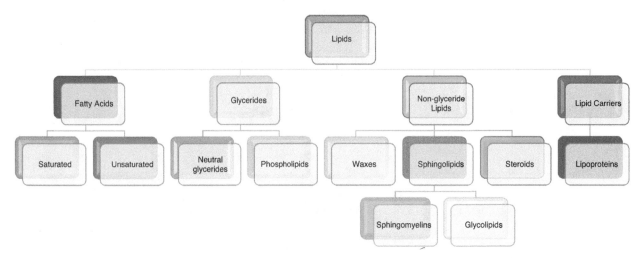

Figure 4.1: **Classification of Biologically Important Lipids.** These four classes of lipids—the fatty acids, glycerides, non-glyceride lipids and lipid carriers are the ones we will consider in this book. All of these types of lipids can take part in metabolic processes.

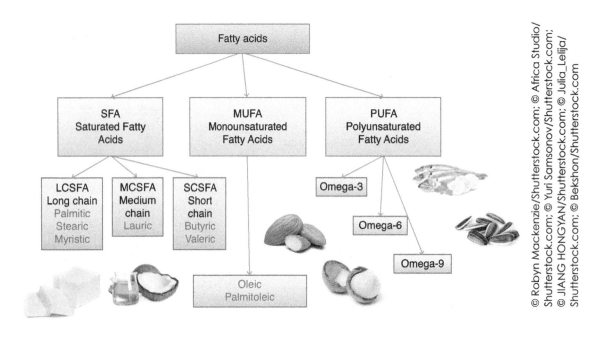

© Robyn Mackenzie/Shutterstock.com; © Africa Studio/Shutterstock.com; © Yuri Samsonov/Shutterstock.com; © JIANG HONGYAN/Shutterstock.com; © Julia_Lelija/Shutterstock.com; © Bekshon/Shutterstock.com

Figure 4.2: **Types of Fatty Acids.** Fatty acids can be subdivided into saturated, monounsaturated, and polyunsaturated forms. Some foods containing these forms are shown below. Butter contains long chain fatty acids, such as palmitic, stearic, and myristic acids. Coconut oil is a good source of lauric acid. Butyric acid is found in butter, while valeric acid is from the plant, Valeriana officinalis, and is usually used as a food additive. Almonds are a good source of oleic acid, while palmitoleic acid can be found in macadamia nuts. Omega 3s are high in fatty fish such as mackerel, while sunflower seeds are a good source of both omega 6 and omega 9 fatty acids.

acids without double bonds can stack on top of one another. On the other hand, the unsaturated fatty acids commonly have kinks and are more loosely packed with one another in a food. An additional interesting point to consider is that saturated fats are solid room temperature, whereas unsaturated fatty acids are liquid at room temperature. Consider butter or lard (high in saturated fat) vs. olive oil (high in monounsaturated fat).

Unsaturated fatty acids can be divided into cis- and trans- structures which refer to the position of the hydrogen atoms in the molecule (Figure 4.3). In the cis-structures, there is both a hydrophilic (polar, likes water) and hydrophobic (non-polar, non-water loving) end, as each of the single hydrogen atoms next to a carbon double bond stick out on the same side of the chain. With the double bond in the cis-conformation, the structure of the fatty acid can be rigid, and can cause a lower melting temperature of the fat due to its rigidity. In the trans conformation, which rarely occurs in nature (small amounts are found naturally in some meat and dairy products, produced by ruminants such as cows, sheep, and goats) but rather is the result of food processing by hydrogenation, the two hydrogens lie on opposite sides of the carbon chain. This allows for slightly less rigidity for the molecule overall, with structures similar to straight saturated fatty acids.

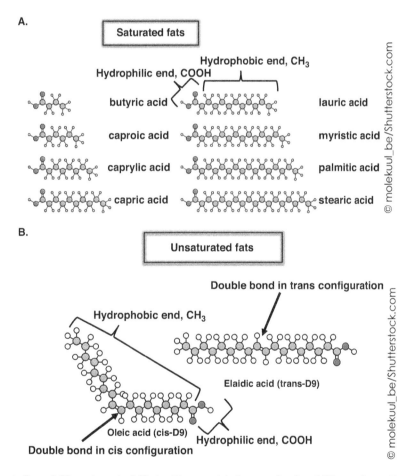

Figure 4.3: **Saturated and Unsaturated Fats**: Fatty acids have a hydrophilic carboxylic end (COOH, shown with red oxygen molecules) and a hydrophobic end (linear ending with CH₃ moiety). **(A)** Saturated fats contain no double bonded carbons, and are linear. **(B)** Unsaturated fats have at least one double bond, and can come in the cis or trans configuration. In the trans configuration, the hydrogens are on opposite sides of the molecule, making it linear, like saturated fats. In the cis configuration, hydrogens are on the same side, and there is a kink in the structure. These molecules are more rigid.

Free fatty acids (FFA) are also called non-esterified fatty acids, or NEFA. Fatty acids are attached to a glycerol molecule with an ester bond, so a non-esterified fatty acid is one, that is not attached with an ester bond to a glycerol molecule. These non-food-bound fatty acids are found in plasma at concentrations up to 1 mM, and are bound to the blood protein albumin. Take a look at Figure 4.2, which shows the types of saturated (SFA), MUFA, and PUFA molecules, as well as common food sources.

Giving Fats a Name

Unfortunately for students trying to grasp metabolism, scientists in the metabolism field (and most other fields as well!) have developed multiple names for processes, proteins, and molecules (think TCA cycle, Krebs Cycle, Citric Acid Cycle, etc). Fatty acid names were not immune to this problem. The currently accepted fatty acid nomenclature rules allow us to distinguish between chain length and number of double bonds. The Delta (Δ) system denotes chain length, and number of double bonds, as well as the positions of all double bonds. The other system, called the Omega (ω) system gives the chain length, number of double bonds, and the position of the first double bond from the methyl (CH_3) end (Figure 4.4). Then there are scientific names, as well as so-called "trivial" names. Let's take a look at how we name a common fatty acid, linoleic acid. As shown in Figure 4.4, when the delta system is used, we would call the acid 18:2 $\Delta^{9,12}$. For the omega system, we would call linoleic acid 18:2 ω-6 (this one would sometimes also be notated as 18:2 n-6). The trivial name for linoleic acid is "linoleic acid" (of course), while the scientific name is 9, 12-octadecadienoic acid. To break down the scientific name, you can see that they are a combination of Latin terms for numbers (octo = 8, and deca = 10, so "18"), with the rest the chemical name for the fatty acid. Why do you need to know this? Because in the scientific literature, the trivial, scientific, delta, and omega names are used interchangeably—or perhaps one author will stick to one form, while another, referring to exactly the same fatty acid, will use a different nomenclature. That makes things tricky but not impossible if you understand how the

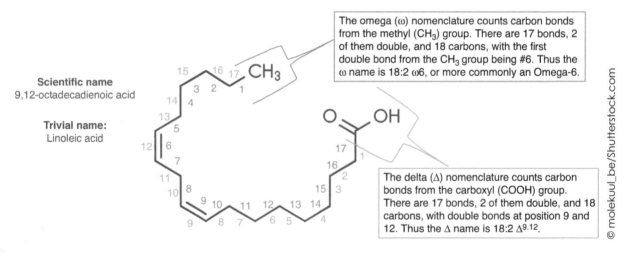

Figure 4.4: **Naming conventions:** This example shows linoleic acid, which is the so-called trivial name for the fatty acid. The scientific name is 9,12-octadecadienoic acid. The omega and delta naming conventions are explained in the graphic.

Table 4.1: **Nomenclature for common essential and non-essential fatty acids.** The essential fatty acids cannot be synthesized by the body and must be obtained from foods.

Notation	Common Name	Formula	Essential or Nonessential
Saturated Fatty Acids			
14:0	Myristic acid	$CH_3\text{-}(CH_2)_{12}\text{-}COOH$	nonessential
16:0	Palmitic acid	$CH_3\text{-}(CH_2)_{14}\text{-}COOH$	nonessential
18:0	Stearic acid	$CH_3\text{-}(CH_2)_{16}\text{-}COOH$	nonessential
20:0	Arachidic acid	$CH_3\text{-}(CH_2)_{18}\text{-}COOH$	nonessential
22:0	Lignoceric acid	$CH_3\text{-}(CH_2)_{22}\text{-}COOH$	nonessential
Unsaturated Fatty Acids			
16:1 Δ^9 (ω7)	Palmitoleic acid	$CH_3\text{-}(CH_2)_5\text{-}CH{=}CH(CH_2)_7\text{-}COOH$	nonessential
18:1 Δ^9 (ω9)	Oleic acid	$CH_3\text{-}(CH_2)_7\text{-}CH{=}CH(CH_2)_7\text{-}COOH$	nonessential
18:2 $\Delta^{9,12}$ (ω6)	Linoleic acid	$CH_3\text{-}(CH_2)_4\text{-}CH{=}CH\text{-}CH_2\text{-}CH_2)_4\text{-}$ $CH{=}CH\text{-}(CH2)_7\text{-}COOH$	essential
18:3 $\Delta^{9,12,15}$ (ω3)	α-linolenic acid (ALA)	$CH_3\text{-}(CH_2\text{-}CH{=}CH)_3\text{-}(CH_2)_7\text{-}COOH$	essential
20:4 $\Delta^{5,8,11,15}$ (ω6)	Arachidonic acid	$CH_3\text{-}(CH_2)_3\text{-}(CH_2\text{-}CH{=}CH)_4\text{-}(CH_2)_3\text{-}COOH$	Conditionally essential (if lack of linoleic acid)
20:5 $\Delta^{5,8,11,14,17}$ (ω3)	Eicosapentaenoic acid (EPA)	$CH_3\text{-}(CH_2\text{-}CH{=}CH)_5\text{-}(CH_2)_3\text{-}COOH$	Conditionally essential (if lack of α-linolenic acid)
22:6 $\Delta^{4,7,10,13,16,19}$ (ω3)	Docosahexaenoic acid (DHA)	$CH_3\text{-}(CH_2\text{-}CH{=}CH)_6\text{-}(CH_2)_2\text{-}COOH$	Conditionally essential (if lack of α-linolenic acid)

nomenclature is derived (and remember you can tell which nomenclature is being used by seeing the ω or the Δ, or the Latin names, or nothing).

Take a look at the table (Table 4.1), which lists common, naturally occurring saturated and unsaturated fatty acids with their common names, chemical formulas, and nomenclatures.

Essentially Fat.... the Essential and Non-essential Fatty Acids

Fatty acids can be divided into those that are non-essential and those that are essential. What's the difference? The essential ones must be taken in via diet, while the non-essential can be synthesized in our body—we need all of these fatty acids, but the terminology refers to whether we can make it, or need it in our diet. For the essential fatty acids, plants, and fish, for example have the enzymes necessary to make these types of fatty acids, which means that they have the ability to synthesize fatty acids with double bonds beyond the C-9 bond, which humans do not. As shown on Table 4.1, α-linolenic acid is one of these essential fatty acids, and it does indeed have double bonds at positions 9, 12, and 15. Docosahexaenoic acid (DHA) can be obtained by eating fatty fish, like salmon, and while humans and other animals can synthesize both DHA and eicosapentaeonic acid (EPA), we are less efficient at doing that for DHA, and their synthesis requires the substrate α-linolenic acid, to be in abundance. Thus, these are considered "conditionally" essential, and most individuals try to get these from diet[2]. Arachidonic acid is another "conditionally" essential fatty acid. It is synthesized from the omega-6, linoleic acid, but is also commonly found in food.

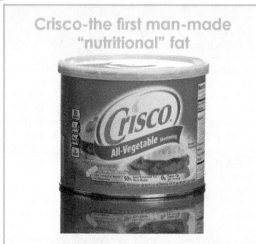

Crisco-the first man-made "nutritional" fat

A scientist at Proctor and Gamble developed Crisco™ shortening, which was the first trans-fat made for consumption by humans. According to an article in the LA Times, it was originally intended as a lard replacement for making soap, and the name is derived from "crystalized cottonseed oil".[3]

Trans fats cannot be synthesized in our bodies, but are not essential either. Some trans fatty acids occur naturally, but many of these were synthesized and commercially produced for use in manufactured foods. Why? Because the chemical structure of a trans-fatty acid can sometimes increase the shelf life, reduce susceptibility to heat, and increase overall stability of the fatty acid. Take a look back at Figure 4.3, and you can see that the overall structure of a trans fatty acid is different, when compared to the associated cis fatty acid. This is because the way to make a trans fatty acid is by adding in hydrogens and breaking some of the double bonds. This process, called hydrogenation, has been used for over 100 years now by many different food scientists as a way that was thought to be beneficial (by providing more stable oils). However, many of these trans fats (but not all) have been found to associated with negative health outcomes (increased 'bad' cholesterol transporters (LDL) and decreased 'good' cholesterol transporters (HDL), more later on this), and the US government now requires special labeling for foods containing trans fatty acids and are banning them completely by the end of 2018.

Sugary-lipids—the Glycerolipids

Many of the fatty acids that were discussed above, at least the naturally occurring ones, are actually found in the form of glycerolipids or acylglycerols. These are mono-, di-, and triesters of a glycerol (hence the reference to "sugary" in the section title, remember from earlier that glycerol is made from glucose?) with their associated fatty acids (Figure 4.5). They can be metabolized in our bodies to release fatty acids for use in metabolism (energy production). The most common glycerolipid is a triacylgycerol or TAG (also referred to as simply triglyceride). TAGs represent highly concentrated energy storage, and as we'll see later in this chapter, the free fatty acids from TAGs can enter beta-oxidation and produce many ATP molecules. TAGs are transported in lipoproteins within our bloodstream. As they can be composed of either saturated or unsaturated fatty acids they can either be in a solid,

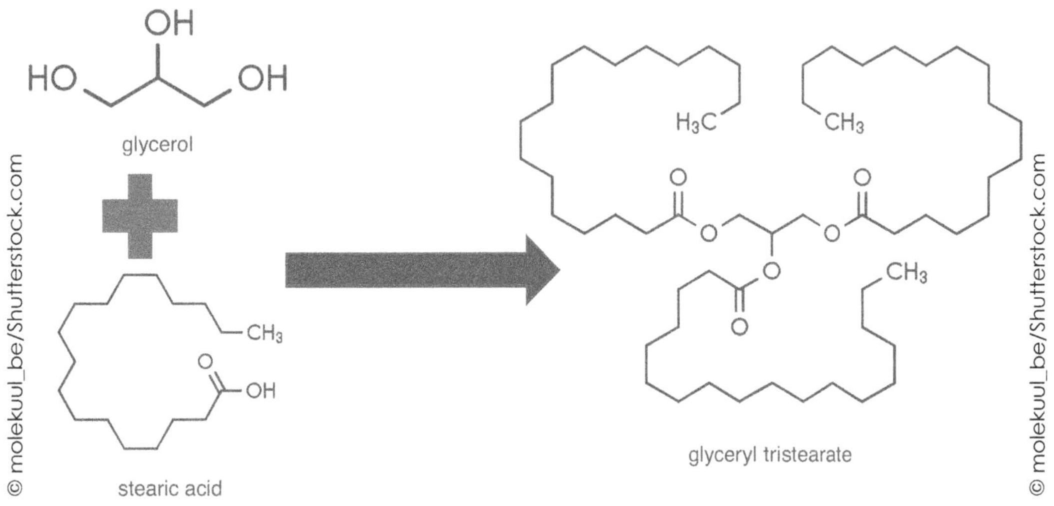

Figure 4.5: Glycerolipids. Glycerolipids are composed of a glycerol molecule and one or more fatty acid molecules. In this example, one glycerol molecules and three molecules of the saturated fatty acid stearic acid are formed into a triacylglycerol or triglyceride, known as glyceryl tristearate.

semi-solid, or liquid form (we discussed this earlier). In fact, most of the stored body fat in our bodies is in the form of TAGs.

Sterols

Sterols are characterized by a four-ring core structure, called a cyclopentanoperhydrophenanthrene core—whew—let's just call this the sterol core (Figure 4.6). While the free form of cholesterol can exist, it can also be conjugated to a fatty acid, and is transported in lipoproteins. Cholesterol is the only sterol made by animals, while plants can make other types of sterols, which are usually called phytosterols. There is significant evidence from a number of published, peer-reviewed articles that ingestion of phytosterols such as sitosterol and campesterol, can block absorption of animal-based cholesterol (e.g.[4]). However, increased dietary cholesterol can raise serum cholesterol levels in adults, although the amount of increase differs widely between individuals[5]. Even so, we need cholesterol, as it serves as a precursor for the production of bile acids, steroid hormones such as testosterone, adrenocortical steroid hormones, and as the building block for the production of Vitamin D in our skin[6]. In addition, removal of cholesterol from the diet increases liver production of cholesterol, and there are studies showing that

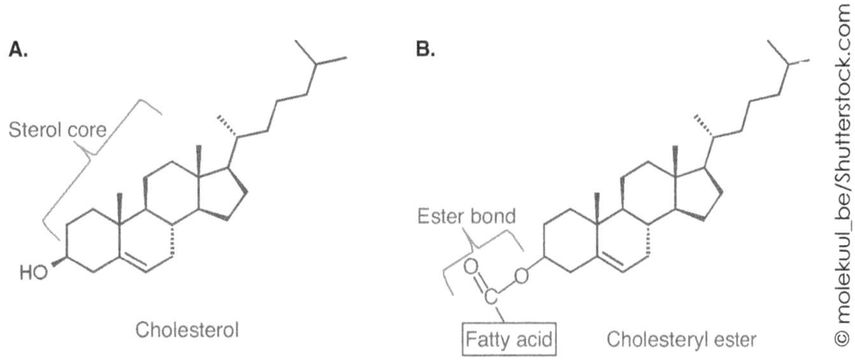

Figure 4.6: Sterols The only sterol made by animals is the cholesterol molecule (**A**). When a fatty acid is attached, via an ester bond, the cholesterol molecule becomes a cholesteryl ester (**B**).

serum cholesterol levels are fine-tuned in some individuals such that even ingesting a high cholesterol diet does not result in much of a change in serum cholesterol levels, due to the downregulation of the rate-limiting enzyme HMG CoA Reductase (more about this enzyme in a later chapter)[5].

Phospholipids

As their name implies, phospholipids are a group of lipids that at least have a phosphate group. These phospholipids are often found in our cell membranes where they are involved in various cellular signaling events. The structure of phospholipids is such that it looks like a ball on a stick—with the "head" being composed of a phosphorylated glycerol group with a head group like choline or inositol, and the stick being composed of two specific fatty acids. When the molecules are organized to all face in the same direction, and doubled up, as shown in Figure 4.7, a very unique structure can be built—the cell or organelle membrane. The interesting and unique feature of cell and organelle membranes is that they have both hydrophobic (i.e. the fatty acid tails) which point inwards, and hydrophilic regions (the phosphoglycerol head group) which are on the outside. Some common phospholipids that are found in animal cell membranes include phosphatidylcholine, phosphatidylserine, phosphatidylinositol, and phosphatidylethanolamine (Figure 4.7A). Sphingolipids (also called sphingophosphatides) are classified within the non-glycerol lipids, but are phospholipids that have an amino alcohol group at their core derived from a serine amino acid, a phosphate, and fatty acids.[7] The most common sphingolipids found in cell membranes are sphingomyelin (Figure 4.7B). Sphingolipids also appear to interact with cholesterol in cell membranes, forming lipid rafts, which gives structure and rigidity to the cell membrane.

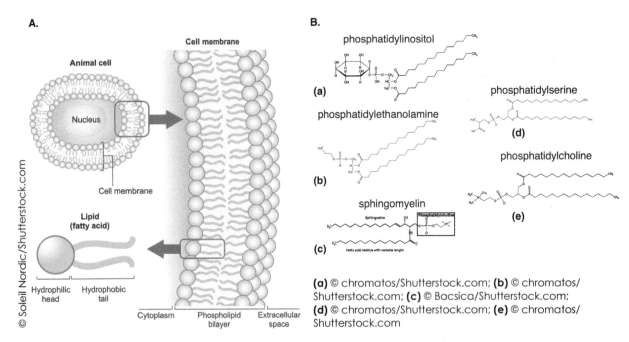

(a) © chromatos/Shutterstock.com; **(b)** © chromatos/Shutterstock.com; **(c)** © Bacsica/Shutterstock.com; **(d)** © chromatos/Shutterstock.com; **(e)** © chromatos/Shutterstock.com

Figure 4.7: **Phospholipids for membranes (A)** As shown, a phospholipid is composed of a phosphorylated glycerol molecule, with a fatty acid tail. The tail can be made of either saturated fats (in which case it may be straight and make the membrane somewhat rigid, or unsaturated fats, which would make the membrane more fluid- they disrupt the tightly packed saturated fatty acids). **(B)** The most common phospholipids found in cell membranes are phosphatidylcholine, phosphatidylserine, phosphatidylethanolamine, and phosphatidylinositol. One can also have sphingolipids in the cell membrane, such as ceramide which is used to form sphingomyelin. Sphingolipids have an amino (NH_3) backbone derived from serine (instead of a glycerol backbone), along with the fatty acids, a phosphate group, and a head group.

Lipoproteins

We'll talk about proteins in the next chapter, but it is important to consider lipoproteins here with the lipids. Lipoproteins were first isolated from horse serum in the 1920's, as an acid-precipitable complex containing 59.1% protein, 22.7% phospholipids, and 17.9% cholesterol esters[8]. In later studies, lipoproteins were divided into α- and β-lipoproteins, in which the β-lipoproteins were generally higher in molecular weight, but the α-lipoproteins had lower lipid and higher protein contents[8]. Ultracentrifugation techniques led to the further classification based on floatation in salt gradients with the density of chylomicrons < very-low density lipoproteins (VLDL) < low-density lipoproteins (LDL) < high-density lipoproteins (HDL). As shown on Figure 4.8A this differential density of lipoproteins is due to the different composition of each type of lipoprotein, in terms of the percent of triglycerides, cholesterol, phospholipids, and proteins. Looking a little more closely (Figure 4.8B), we can see that the general structure of the lipoprotein is made up of a cholesterol and triglyceride core, with a phospholipid membrane containing pro-

> ## Genetics of hypercholesterolemia
>
> Familial hypercholesterolemia, or high cholesterol levels that are inherited within families and related to variations in specific genes, are a major cause of high cholesterol and cardiovascular disease in the general population. In a recent study, three separate genes, the LDL-receptor, the APOB gene (part of chylomicrons and low density lipoproteins) and the PCSK9 gene (an enzyme that appears to break down LDL receptors and control cholesterol) were linked to high cholesterol levels in individuals[7]. As we identify more genes and understand their biological functions we may be able to help individuals with these types of metabolic disorders.

teins inserted in the membrane. These proteins are lipid-binding proteins that form a larger protein family called apolipoproteins. Apolipoprotein B is the primary protein within the lower density lipoproteins—namely chylomicrons, VLDLs, and LDLs. The other apolipoproteins (e.g. ApoA, ApoC, ApoE, etc), are generally found on HDLs, although they can be found in smaller amounts on the other lipoproteins. Generally, the apolipoprotein components of lipoproteins help to maintain structure, but can also have enzymatic, and receptor-binding activities[8], which will be talked about in later chapters.

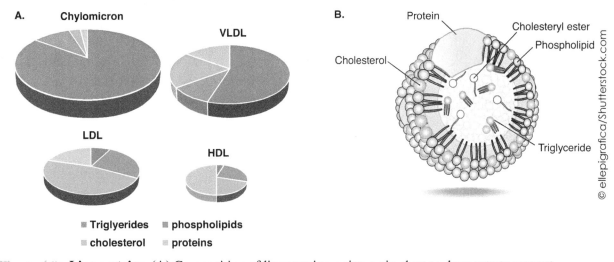

Figure 4.8: Lipoproteins. (A) Composition of lipoproteins, using a pie-chart to demonstrate percent of triglycerides, phospholipids, cholesterol and proteins in each type. Note that the size difference from chylomicrons (the largest) > very low density lipoproteins (VLDLs) > low density lipoproteins (LDLs) > high density lipoproteins (HDLs), which are the smallest. **(B)** Cartoon drawing of a representative serum lipoprotein.

Let's Burn this Fat!

Any tissue in the body that has mitochondria has the ability to store TAGs, making TAGs a great source of stored energy. This isn't true for glycogen, the stored form for sugars specific to the liver and muscle, which means that TAGs are a universal energy source for all tissues. While this is a "good" thing, in principal, with the increases in obesity these days, storage of excess TAGs in some tissues can have pathologic consequences, such as metabolic disease—more on that in a later chapter. Fat metabolism encompasses the synthesis, storage, transport, and oxidation of lipids, and depends on the location of the fats, as well as the metabolic condition of the individual.

As we absorb fatty acids or cholesterol in our diet, these molecules are re-synthesized into TAGs and cholesterol esters in our enterocytes, absorptive cells in the small intestine, which incorporate them into chylomicrons where they are transported around the body. When we are in the fed state (meaning just after eating a meal), fatty acids are also directly synthesized from glucose sources, as we saw previously in a state of excess carbohydrate intake. *De novo* fatty acid synthesis in the liver produces fatty acids that are synthesized into TAGs and can be released into circulation in a VLDL. In the fasted state (at least 6 or more after our last meal), fatty acids are released from adipocytes, and transported bound to albumin, and are picked up by cells that metabolize them for energy, especially skeletal muscle.

Generally, fatty acids are stored by converting them into TAGs which can later be released and used as described above. This is important to tissues such as skeletal muscles which sometimes need to have immediate access to metabolizable energy, using a process called lipolysis (we will describe this more later).

Once the free fatty acid is liberated from the TAG, entry of the fatty acid into the mitochondria is regulated. For example, to get into the mitochondria, the free fatty acid receives a CoA moiety, becoming an acyl CoA, at the equivalent expense of 2 ATP (1 ATP $\rightarrow$ AMP), which can be used in beta oxidation to produce acetyl CoAs and reducing equivalents (FADH$_2$ and NADH). Let's look at this process in a little more detail.

Short chain fatty acids can get into the mitochondria directly, although they still need to have a CoA moiety attached, and the enzyme acyl CoA synthetase does the job in the matrix of the mitochondria[9] (Figure 4.9). Once activated, they can begin beta oxidation. Longer chain fatty acyl CoAs enter through the outer mitochondrial membrane via a protein complex[10]. One of the proteins in the complex is carnitine palmitoyltransferase I (CPT1). The CoA molecule is not permeable to the inner mitochondrial membrane and therefore is swapped out for a carnitine molecule. (Carnitine is made up of methionine and lysine and is synthesized in the liver and kidneys.) It is still not yet clear whether the fatty acyl-carnitine is formed in the cytosol or in the intermembrane space. Once in the intermembrane space, the fatty acyl-carnitine still needs to use a specialized transport system to get through the inner membrane—mainly the protein transporter: carnitine acylcarnitine translocase (SLC25A20). There a second CPT enzyme, embedded on the matrix side of the inner membrane (conveniently called CPT II) that removes the carnitine and re-attaches a CoA , and now the fatty acyl-CoA can enter the beta oxidation process[9]. This process of getting fatty acids into the mitochondria using a carnitine molecule is called the carnitine transport system, or carnitine shuttle.

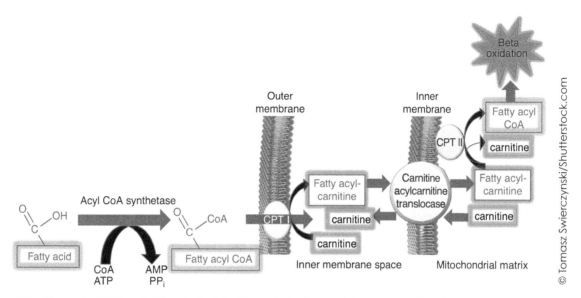

Figure 4.9: **Fatty Acid Metabolism in brief.** Short chain fatty acids can pass directly into the mitochondrial matrix and are activated there. Longer chain fatty acids are activated in the cytoplasm by acyl CoA synthetase. LCFAs then pass through the outer membrane via a protein complex including carnitine palmitoyltransferase 1 (CPT1), which conjugates a carnitine in exchange for the CoA. The fatty acyl-carnitine is then transported through the inner membrane through the protein transporter, carnitine acylcarnitine translocase. Once inside the matrix, CPTII exchanges the carnitine for a CoA and now beta-oxidation can begin. The carnitine acylcarnitine translocase protein is an antiport exchanging the fatty acyl-carnitine for a carnitine molecule.

Beta oxidation occurs within the mitochondrial matrix, and yields one $FADH_2$, one NADH and one acetyl CoA molecule for each turn of the cycle (Figure 4.10). In other words, each two-carbon cleavage from the carboxy end of the fatty acid are used to form another molecule of acetyl CoA which can go directly into the TCA cycle generating 10 ATPs (remember this from earlier?). The process also generates an $FADH_2$ and an NADH for the electron transport chain, which gives 1.5 and 2.5 more ATPs respectively (for a total of 4 more). What this means is that a lot of energy (ATP) can be formed from beta oxidation of fatty acids. For example, if we use the 16-carbon palmitic fatty acid in beta oxidation, we can calculate the ATP generated. Palmitic acid is 16 carbons long and acetyl CoA is two carbons long. As the fatty acid goes through each cycle of beta oxidation, two carbons are removed at a time producing 1 acetyl CoA. So, to determine the amount of acetyl CoAs produced, you take the carbon number divided by 2: 16/2 = 8 acetyl CoAs. Next, knowing that each cycle of beta oxidation produces 1 NADH and 1 $FADH_2$, we need to know the number of beta oxidation cycles. We take the fatty acid carbon number and divide it again by 2, but we subtract 1 cycle because the last cycle produces 2 acetyl CoAs: 16/2 −1 = 7 cycles. Therefore, the following net ATPs are generated:

7 cycles (carbon-carbon cleavages) → 7 × 4 = 28 ATP (from NADH and $FADH_2$ formation)
8 acetyl CoA molecules generated → 8 × 10 = 80 ATP (produced from the TCA cycle)
TOTAL produced → 28 + 80 = 108 ATPs
2 ATP equivalents used for activation (adding the CoA) −2
NET produced →106 ATPs

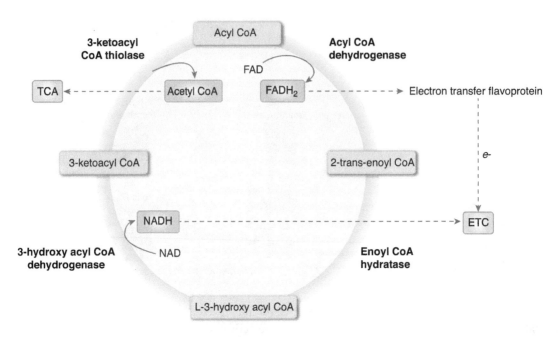

Figure 4.10:   **Beta Oxidation.** Fatty acyl CoA molecules go through a cyclic degradation, with each cycle producing acetyl CoA for the TCA cycle, and $FADH_2$ and NADH which can go directly into the electron transport chain.

Compared to a single glucose molecule, which will give 30–32 ATPs, a single fat molecule packs a lot more energy, right? As palmitic acid is the most abundant saturated fatty acid stored in adipose tissue, and the most abundant in the body[11], there can be a lot of stored energy for an individual to use if and when it is needed.

What about the oxidation of an unsaturated fatty acid? Unsaturated fatty acids also use beta oxidation. However, the second enzyme in beta oxidation-enoyl CoA hydratase needs a trans double bond. As you may remember most unsaturated fatty acids are in the cis-conformation. So, an unsaturated fatty acid skips the first step of beta oxidation and a special isomerase enzyme (enoyl CoA isomerase) converts the cis to a trans double bond if the bond is located on an odd-numbered carbon (ex. when the double bond is between C9 and C10). Because of this, the production of 1 $FADH_2$ is missed, reducing the ATP yield by 1.5 ATP. For polyunsaturated fatty acids, not only do we need the enoyl CoA isomerase enzyme to convert the cis bonds into trans bonds, a second enzyme, 2,4-dienoyl reductase (and NADPH), is needed when the double bond is located on an even-numbered carbon. In this situation, the double bond is handled by the isomerase and the reductase together. For each cis double bond present, there is a reduction of ATP potential by 1.5, due to the loss of $FADH_2$ production in the first enzymatic step of beta oxidation.

What about odd-chained fatty acids? The odd-chain fatty-acids are oxidized during beta-oxidation, just like even-chained fatty acids. The only difference is in the final cycle, where instead of 2 acetyl CoAs produced, your final products are an acetyl CoA and a propionyl CoA. Propionyl CoA can be converted to succinyl CoA in three enzymatic steps, via propionyl CoA carboxylase

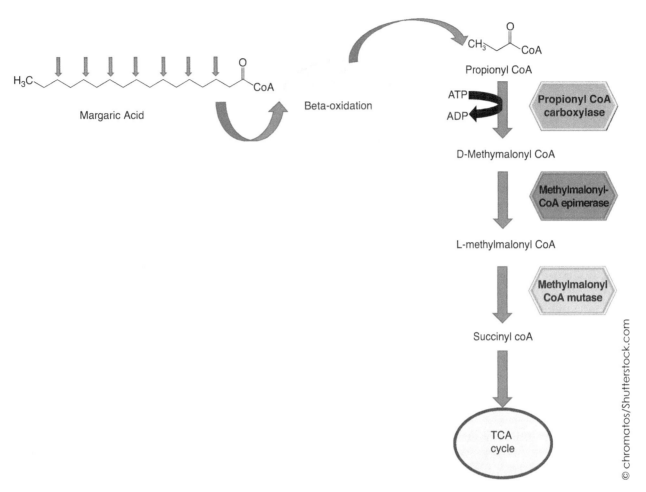

Figure 4.11: **Odd Chain Beta Oxidation.** Odd chain Fatty acyl CoA molecules go through beta oxidation, with each cycle producing acetyl CoA for the TCA cycle, and FADH$_2$ and NADH which can go directly into the electron transport cycle. The last cycle produces one acetyl CoA and one propionyl CoA. Margaric acid (heptadecanoic acid) is shown as an example which would go through 7 rounds of beta oxidation (shown by arrows), making 7 acetyl CoA molecules, 7 FADH$_2$ molecules and 7 NADH molecules, along with one propionyl CoA. The propionyl CoA is further degraded to succinyl CoA as shown, using one ATP molecule.

(using biotin and 1 ATP), methylmalonyl CoA racemase, and methylmalonyl CoA mutase (using B12), and can then enter the TCA cycle (Figure 4.11). Succinyl CoA skips the first 3 enzymatic steps of the TCA cycle, thereby missing the production of 2 NADH (5 ATP). For instance, if you had margaric acid (17:0), you would have 7 acetyl CoAs and 1 succinyl CoA. There would be 7 cycles, so your ATP yield would be:

7 cycles (carbon-carbon cleavages) → 7 × 4 = 28 ATP (from NADH and FADH$_2$ formation)
7 acetyl CoA molecules generated → 7 × 10 = 70 ATP (produced from the TCA cycle)

1 succinyl CoA → 1 × 5 = 5 ATP (produced from the TCA cycle) – 1 ATP invested = 4 ATP
TOTAL produced → 28 + 70 + 4 = 102 ATPs
2 ATP equivalents used for activation (adding the CoA) –2
NET produced → 100 ATPs

The production of ATP for this odd chain fatty acid which has the same number of beta oxidation cycles as the smaller 16:0 palmitic acid, is actually less. Calculate it and see for yourself!

Summary

Fats and water do not mix, and because of this fact, lipids are handled in a special way by our bodies. As we've seen in this chapter, glyceride and non-glyceride lipids travel in specialized lipoproteins such as chylomicrons or VLDLs, free fatty acids travel bound to albumin, and both need to be transported into cells and into mitochondria using specialized systems. Lipids, namely the fatty acids, also have their own cyclic pathway for releasing energy—beta oxidation which yields boatloads of energy for the body. The structure of lipids—especially phospholipids, cholesterol, and glycolipids, make them important components of cell membranes, and useful in making steroid hormones, including Vitamin D, for our body.

Points to ponder

➢ Can you calculate ATP amounts that would come from different types of fatty acids (without looking back at the book chapter)? Compare even- and odd-numbered fatty acid ATP generation.

➢ Vitamin D needs cholesterol to be synthesized by our bodies, and surprisingly circulating Vitamin D levels are generally low in obese patients. However, according to one article, supplementation of Vitamin D to obese rodents ramped up beta oxidation. Take a look at the article by Marcotorchino and colleagues[12] and see what you think.

➢ Consider what is known about TAGs and other lipids, and the risk of cardiovascular disease. Is this a genetic or environmental component (or both?).

➢ Based on the need for carnitine to get long chain fatty acids into the mitochondria, do you think dietary supplementation with carnitine will increase the body's ability to burn fat? There is actually quite a bit of scientific literature on this topic. Spend some time reading on this topic and see what you find.

References

1. McNaught AD, Wilkinson A. IUPAC. Compendium of Chemical Terminology, 2nd ed. (the "Gold Book"). 1997; http://goldbook.iupac.org/html/F/F02330.html. Accessed February 28, 2018.

2. Muskiet FA, Fokkema MR, Schaafsma A, Boersma ER, Crawford MA. Is docosahexaenoic acid (DHA) essential? Lessons from DHA status regulation, our ancient diet, epidemiology and randomized controlled trials. *J Nutr.* 2004;134(1):183–186.

3. Hallock B. Rise and fall of trans fat: A history of partially hydrogenated oil. In. *Los Angeles Times.* Los Angeles 2013.

4. Gylling H, Plat J, Turley S, et al. Plant sterols and plant stanols in the management of dyslipidaemia and prevention of cardiovascular disease. *Atherosclerosis.* 2014;232(2):346–360.
5. Grundy SM. Does Dietary Cholesterol Matter? *Curr Atheroscler Rep.* 2016;18(11):68.
6. Gault CR, Obeid LM, Hannun YA. An overview of sphingolipid metabolism: from synthesis to breakdown. *Adv Exp Med Biol.* 2010;688:1–23.
7. Di Taranto MD, Benito-Vicente A, Giacobbe C, et al. Identification and in vitro characterization of two new PCSK9 Gain of Function variants found in patients with Familial Hypercholesterolemia. *Sci Rep.* 2017;7(1):15282.
8. Alaupovic P. Significance of apolipoproteins for structure, function, and classification of plasma lipoproteins. *Methods Enzymol.* 1996;263:32–60.
9. Lundsgaard AM, Fritzen AM, Kiens B. Molecular Regulation of Fatty Acid Oxidation in Skeletal Muscle during Aerobic Exercise. *Trends Endocrinol Metab.* 2018;29(1):18–30.
10. Console L, Giangregorio N, Indiveri C, Tonazzi A. Carnitine/acylcarnitine translocase and carnitine palmitoyltransferase 2 form a complex in the inner mitochondrial membrane. *Mol Cell Biochem.* 2014;394(1–2):307–314.
11. Kokatnur MG, Oalmann MC, Johnson WD, Malcom GT, Strong JP. Fatty acid composition of human adipose tissue from two anatomical sites in a biracial community. *Am J Clin Nutr.* 1979;32(11):2198–2205.
12. Marcotorchino J, Tourniaire F, Astier J, et al. Vitamin D protects against diet-induced obesity by enhancing fatty acid oxidation. *J Nutr Biochem.* 2014;25(10):1077–1083.

CHAPTER 5

Macronutrient metabolism: Breaking Down Proteins

Proteins are the workhorses of the cell—messengers, builders, designers and regulators. As shown in Table 5.1, there are 20 standard amino acids that vertebrates use to make proteins. Note that there are a lot of ways that we name these amino acids—by full name, by three-letter abbreviation, and by single letter abbreviation. Each amino acid is encoded by a three letter RNA code (a codon), and in some cases, multiple RNA codes will signify the same single amino acid (see box). Note that there are actually 23 known amino acids—two of which are selenocysteine (Sec/U) and selenomethione, in which there is a selenium molecule instead of the sulfur group on the side chain of the amino acids, and the third being pyrrolysine (Pyr/O), which has a pyrroline ring as part of the side chain of lysine. Only selenocysteine is made in vertebrates. Selenomethionine is made by plants and can be ingested by humans to get the selenium micronutrient, while pyrrolysine is only in some bacterial species.

In addition to their names, Table 5.2 shows that we can classify amino acids by net electrical charge (positive, negative, and neutral), structure (i.e. presence or absence of a ring in their side chains), polarity (i.e. whether they can interact with water), and their need in the body (whether they are essential—which means we cannot make them, conditionally essential—which means we may need them depending on other

Amino acid codons

To find an amino acid codon, start in the center of the wheel (5') and move outwards to pick the first, second, and third nucleotide of the codon (outer circle, 3'). Note that in some cases, amino acids can share the same second nucleotide, but have one of the four unique third nucleotides. Some amino acids, such as methionine (the start codon for proteins) have only one codon, whereas others, such as proline, are encoded by four different codons. There are also three "stop" codons that tell the ribosome to stop translation of the mRNA.

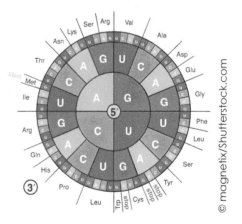

© magnetix/Shutterstock.com

Did you know?

Selenocysteine is used to make selenoproteins such as glutathione peroxidase and thioredoxin reductase, both of which are key to free-radical neutralization.

Table 5.1: The Amino Acids. Separated by essential, conditionally essential, and non-essential. Side chain categories and abbreviations are also shown.

Amino Acid Type Essential (we don't make enough of these)	Abbreviation 3 letter/ Single letter	Side Chains Aliphatic Hydroxy Sulfur Acidic Basic Aromatic Imino
Histidine	His/H	Basic
Isoleucine	Ile/I	Aliphatic
Leucine	Leu/L	Aliphatic
Methionine	Met/M	Sulfur
Phenylalanine	Phe/F	Aromatic
Threonine	Thr/T	Hydroxyl
Tryptophan	Trp/W	Aromatic
Valine	Val/V	Aliphatic
Lysine	Lys/K	Basic

Amino Acid Type Conditionally essential (we can make these but sometimes need more)	Abbreviation 3 letter/ Single letter	Side Chains Aliphatic Hydroxy Sulfur Acidic Basic Aromatic Imino
Arginine	Arg/R	Basic
Asparagine	Asn/N	Acidic
Glutamate	Gln/Q	Acidic
Glycine	Gly/G	Aliphatic
Proline	Pro/P	Imino
Serine	Ser/S	Hydroxyl
Tyrosine	Tyr/Y	Hydroxyl and Aromatic

Amino Acid Type Non-essential (we make lots of these)	Abbreviation 3 letter/ Single letter	Side Chains Aliphatic Hydroxy Sulfur Acidic Basic Aromatic Imino
Alanine	Ala/A	Aliphatic
Aspartate	Asp/D	Acidic
Cysteine	Cys/C	Sulfur
Glutamate	Glu/E	Acidic

Table 5.2: Polarity and Charge of Amino Acids. Separated by essential, conditionally essential, non-essential status.

Essential Amino Acids	Polarity	Charge at pH 7.2	Conditionally essential Amino Acids	Polarity	Charge at pH 7.2	Non-essential Amino Acids	Polarity	Charge at pH 7.2
Histidine	Polar	+ Charged	Arginine	Polar	+ Charged	Alanine	Non-polar	Neutral
Isoleucine	Non-polar	Neutral	Asparagine	Polar	Neutral	Aspartate	Polar	- Charged
Leucine	Non-polar	Neutral	Glutamine	Polar	Neutral	Cysteine	Polar	Neutral
Methionine	Non-polar	Neutral	Glycine	Non-polar	Neutral	Glutamate	Polar	- Charged
Phenylalanine	Non-polar	Neutral	Proline	Non-polar	Neutral			
Threonine	Polar	Neutral	Serine	Polar	Neutral			
Tryptophan	Non-polar	Neutral	Tyrosine	Non-polar	Neutral			
Valine	Non-polar	Neutral						
Lysine	Polar	+ Charged						

factors, or non-essential—which means we can derive them from other building blocks in our body). As shown in Tables 5.1 and 5.2, these classifications result in groupings of the essential, conditionally essential and non-essential amino acids, each containing different amino acid types. Finally, amino acids are also classified by how they are metabolized—for metabolic nutrition, we classify amino acids into ketogenic or glucogenic groups, which tells us about how they are metabolized So, let's talk about the metabolism of amino acids.

Amino Acid Structure and Classification

Our amino acids

All amino acids have a central carbon molecule with at least one amino group (-NH$_3$), one carboxyl group (-COOH), and a side chain (termed an -R group) (Figure 5.1). The R group specifies which amino acid it is—each one has a unique side chain compared to the others. In addition, amino acids can be further classified by their R-groups, which can be divided into aliphatic groups, hydroxyl groups, aromatic ring groups, those containing sulfur molecule, or those that are acidic, basic, or imino (Table 5.1).

Within body fluids amino acids will donate or accept protons (H$^+$) depending on the pH of the solution they are in. At physiological pH, amino acids are predominately di-polar, which means that they have a positive charge at the amino end, and a negative charge at the carboxy end (Figure 5.1). A molecule with a positive and a negative end is also called a "zwitterion". The interesting thing about zwitterions is that they can gain or lose protons, depending on the pH of the environment. For example, in the stomach (a pH of approximately 2), the amino acid would be fully protonated (-NH$_3^+$ and -COOH), while in a basic environment (a pH of 10—however no place in the body has this basic of a pH), amino acids would be fully de-protonated (-NH$_2$ and -COO$^-$). The small intestine has a slightly basic pH of ~8.0, but this is still not basic enough to fully deprotonate amino acids. Amino acids are classified by their charge at physiological pH, which takes into account the amino group, the carboxy group, and the side group charge, to make an overall charge determination (see Table 5.2).

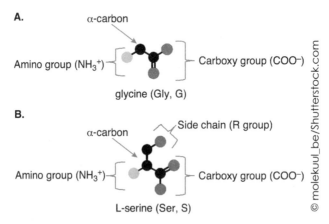

A.
α-carbon
Amino group (NH$_3^+$) — Carboxy group (COO$^-$)
glycine (Gly, G)

B.
Side chain (R group)
α-carbon
Amino group (NH$_3^+$) — Carboxy group (COO$^-$)
L-serine (Ser, S)

© molekuul_be/Shutterstock.com

Figure 5.1: **Amino Acid Structure**. An amino acid always contains an amino group (-NH$_2$, which is protonated at physiological pH to NH$_3$), a carboxy group (-COOH, which is deprotonated at physiological pH to -COO$^-$), and a side chain. In the top example (**A**), which is the simplest amino acid, glycine, the side chain is just a hydrogen attached to the connecting carbon atom. In the bottom example of serine (**B**), the side chain is a methylene group (-CH$_2$) connected to a hydroxyl group (-OH). The alpha carbon (indicated by the arrow) gives the amino acids with side groups chirality, designated as L (levo or left) or D (dextro or right), but in nature, the D-forms of amino acids are rare, and only the L-forms are used to make proteins. (Hydrogen atoms are not shown.)

Side Group Classifications

Let's consider each of these side groups, and their classification in turn. The amino acids containing the aliphatic R-group are glycine, valine, leucine, and isoleucine (Table 5.1). These amino acids are neutral of physiological pH, and only contain carbons and hydrogens in their side chains. In addition, valine, leucine, and isoleucine have branched side chains designating them as branched chain amino acids, which have a different pathway for catabolism/breakdown. This will be discussed in detail later in chapter 12. The amino acids containing hydroxyl groups include serine, threonine, and tyrosine. These amino acids are an important moiety for cellular signaling as the hydroxyl group (-OH) can be exchanged for a phosphate group, when phosphorylated by a kinase, or dephosphorylated back to the -OH group by a phosphatase. Interestingly, tyrosine is also included in the aromatic group of amino acids—or those amino acids that have an aromatic ring as their side group. Phenylalanine and tryptophan are also aromatic amino acids. The aromatic ring in their side group is rather large, making these amino acids perfect components of recognition sites on proteins (think receptors, or enzymatic active sites) for binding to other proteins or molecules.

Sulfur Groups

The next group of amino acids to consider are those whose side groups contain sulfur—methionine and cysteine (Table 5.1). Both of these amino acids are involved in methyl transfer reactions, such part in folate metabolism (Folate or B9 is a micronutrient/vitamin). Cysteine also plays a key role in determining the structure of a protein, as its sulfur atom allows for the formation of di-sulfide bonds between two cysteine amino acids found in different regions of a protein, lending rigidity to an overall protein structure, and helping to facilitate correct protein 3D structure through folding. Methionine is important as the first amino acid added for most protein sequences. Ribosomes scan a mRNA that is ready for translation, and in doing so, recognize the mRNA sequence "AUG" which codes for methionine, letting them know that this is the start codon—a place that they can start translation (building a protein chain).

Acidic and Amide Forms

The next group of amino acids are those that are interchangeable in their formation of acidic and amide forms (Table 5.1). What does this mean? The two amino acids in this group—glutamic acid and aspartic acid, are actually acidic at physiological pH, and as such will provide an overall negative change to proteins containing them. However, when there is a slight switch in their side chain to add an amide group ($-NH_2$), the amino acid takes on its amide form. Glutamine (the amide form of glutamate or glutamic acid) is involved in nitrogen donation for nucleotide synthesis and to maintain acid-base balance in the kidney. Glutamine is formed in the liver when glutamate captures any ammonium ions ($-NH_4$), missed by the urea cycle. Asparagine (the amide form of aspartate or aspartic acid) is a neurotransmitter (glutamate is one too), and when incorporated into proteins, it usually is the terminal amino acid in alpha helical structures of proteins, which helps hold the helical structure, maintaining the overall protein folding, shape and structural integrity.

Charge

The basic amino acids include lysine, arginine, and histidine (Table 5.1). This group of amino acids are positively charged at physiological pH, through an $-NH_2$ in their side chain, which an overall positive (+) charge to the part of the protein they are located in. Lysine is also important as a target of histone protein acetylases (HATs) and deacetylases (HDACs)—and as such, proteins with exposed lysine residues are used for cell signaling.

The last group of amino acids isn't a group at all—rather, it is the single imino amino acid, proline. In addition to being unique for its imino group, which is a five-sided carbon ring, proline is also unique in that it adds rigidity to a protein structure, or it can even put a kink in the protein at the spot where the protein 3D structure needs to transition/change. Of note, proline is hydroxylated in the protein collagen, and when this occurs, the individual collagen chains can intertwine, forming the collage triple helical structure which is part of the extracellular matrix of nearly all of the tissues in our body.

> **Did you know?**
> One group of predominately acetylated proteins are the histones wrapping our DNA. Acetylation can control how tightly or loosely the DNA is wrapped, and contributes to transcriptional control of our genes.

Polarity

We can also group amino acids by their polarity, which simply refers to their affinity (or lack of) for water (Table 5.2). The polar amino acids, and those that are "relatively polar", all help to facilitate solubility and affinity of a protein for water. The more a protein is composed of polar amino acids or is folded so that the polar amino acids are on the outside of the protein, the more likely that it is found in water-type environments, such as the blood or cytosol. Conversely, the non-polar amino acids are going to help the proteins that contain them be localized to waterless environments, such as cell membranes. Proteins are usually composed of both non-polar and polar domains and are folded to expose certain regions along the protein chain, facilitating overall protein function. As you probably guessed already, the side chains for the amino acids determine whether they are polar and/or charged. For example, all of the basic amino acids from Table 5.1 also have a (+) charge at pH 7.2 (Table 5.2). Likewise, most of the acidic amino acids listed on Table 5.1 have a negative charge at pH 7.2, except for glutamine and asparagine, which are both acidic, neutral, and polar. Both glutamine and asparagine have the amide side chains, in which the C=O and NH_2 are uncharged at physiological pH, rendering these acidic amino acids, neutral.

In summary, the amino acids can be classified many different ways, and we can't even group all of one type as being the same group of a second type. In other words, the essential amino acids come in all types, as do the non-essential amino acids. Overall, the composition of proteins containing different percentages of each amino acid, and different properties of the amino acid groups will determine how that protein functions in our bodies. Amino acid composition also determines how the protein is metabolized, and with this knowledge in hand, we can now discuss protein anabolism and catabolism.

Amino Acid Metabolism

As noted above, amino acids can be classified by their fate, in metabolism. That being said, amino acids can be metabolized, producing ketone precursors, glucose precursors, or both. When amino acids are grouped as ketogenic, this does not mean necessarily mean that the amino acid is used for ketones. Rather, it means that the amino acid can be converted to acetyl CoA (a ketone precursor) to enter the TCA cycle (Figure 5.2). There are only two amino acids, leucine and lysine that are

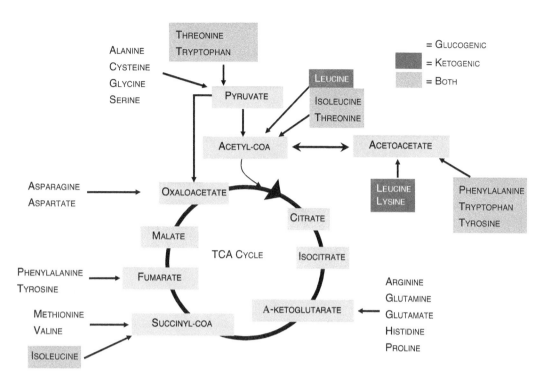

Figure 5.2 **Classification by Fate**. Amino acid side chains determine their catabolic fate and how their carbon skeletons enter the TCA cycle. Ketogenic amino acids are shown in red boxes, while glucogenic amino acids are shown in yellow boxes. Those amino acids whose skeletons are divided in a way that they can undergo both fates are boxed in orange. The entry points to the TCA cycle are indicated by the arrows going to blue-boxed intermediate metabolites.

solely ketogenic, but another five amino acids—phenylalanine, tyrosine, tryptophan, isoleucine, and threonine that can be catabolized both ketogenically or glucogenically. For ketogenic metabolism, many physiological variables determine whether the acetyl CoA from the ketogenic carbon skeletons ends up in the TCA cycle or is eventually made into ketones, and these conditions will be discussed later. Glucogenic amino acids are those amino acids whose carbon skeleton could potentially be converted into glucose. Glucogenic amino acids are converted to alpha keto acids (such as alpha ketoglutarate or oxaloacetate) and then can enter the TCA cycle or they could be converted to glucose via gluconeogenesis, using the substrate pyruvate. Just like ketogenic amino acids, many physiological variables determine if the carbon skeletons of glucogenic amino acids are used for anaplerosis (replenishment of TCA cycle intermediates) or gluconeogenesis. As shown in Figure 5.2, most of the amino acids are glucogenic—only leucine and lysine cannot undergo this catabolic pathway.

Let's talk about isoleucine, leucine, and valine in a little more detail. As you might recall, these three amino acids are grouped into the "branched chain amino acid" (BCAA) subgrouping. All three are also essential amino acids, and in fact comprise up to 40%

Medical fact

Prior to 1982, blood was screened for alanine aminotransferase (ALT) levels as a way to screen out those who might have hepatitis C infections. This is because liver damage (caused by hepatitis C as well as many other things) will result in elevated serum ALT levels. Nowadays, screening for hepatitis C is done using a very sensitive antibody-based test, although ALT levels are still screened to determine if someone has liver damage.

of the essential amino acids that are eaten each day in dietary protein. These branched chain amino acids can only be synthesized by plants, as animals do not have the enzymes necessary for biosynthesis from pyruvate. The branched chain amino acids are essential to maintaining skeletal muscle mass and are catabolized to a greater extent in muscle rather than liver, unlike most of the other amino acids who are mainly catabolized in the liver. In muscle, approximately 70% of the essential amino acids that are broken down are directly recycled into new proteins for muscle[1]. The rest are released and taken up by other tissues. This becomes important, as we will see later on, when an individual is in a fasted state, as the only essential amino acids available for new protein synthesis are those released by protein catabolism[1].

Aminotransferases

The process by which an amino acid can give up its amino group (-NH$_2$) to an alpha-keto acid, leaving us with a keto group and a different amino acid, is called transamination and is catalyzed by aminotransferases (Figure 5.3A). The branched chain amino acids are initially catabolized by the Branched Chain Aminotransferase (BCAT), while Alanine AminoTransferase (ALT) catabolizes alanine, and Aspartate AminoTransferase (AST) catabolizes aspartate (Figure 5.3B). Let's look at these reactions a little more closely. ALT takes the -NH$_2$ amine group from alanine, and puts it onto alpha ketoglutarate, forming glutamate. An alpha keto acid, in this case pyruvate is also formed, and can then enter the TCA cycle via conversion to acetyl CoA through the pyruvate dehydrogenase (PDH) complex (Figure 5.2). Alanine can also be released and circulate in the blood, and when it is picked up by the liver, ALT can also be used to form pyruvate again, the starting material for gluconeogenesis. Alanine is the most commonly used amino acid for gluconeogenesis. These aminotransferase reactions are one of the reasons why alanine and glutamate are non-essential amino acids (Table 5.1).

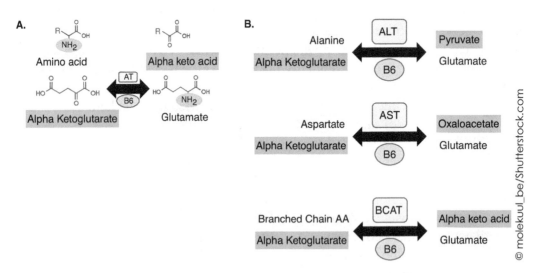

Figure 5.3: **Aminotransferases.** Aminotransferase (AT) reactions. **(A)** Aminotransferases catalyze the transfer of amino groups (-NH$_2$) from an amino acid, to an alpha-keto acid, producing a new amino acid. **(B)** Alanine uses alanine aminotransferase (ALT), and aspartate uses aspartate aminotransferase (AST). All three of the branched chain amino acids are catabolized by branched chain aminotransferase (BCAT). The molecules boxed in blue can enter the TCA cycle or gluconeogenesis (pyruvate), while amino acids are boxed in yellow. The aminotransferase enzymes require the co-enzyme pyridoxal phosphate, a form of Vitamin B6.

AST catalyzes a very similar reaction, by transferring the amine group to alpha-ketoglutarate, forming glutamate and oxaloacetate. This reaction allows for the carbon backbone of aspartate to enter the TCA cycle at oxaloacetate (Figure 5.2). For the branched chain amino acids, the enzyme BCAT takes leucine, isoleucine, or valine, and upon transferring the amine group, $-NH_2$ to alpha-ketoglutarate, forms glutamate and another keto acid (Figure 5.3B). For BCAT, the keto acids formed are different, but all three can be further processed by the Branched Chain Keto Acid Dehydrogenase enzyme (BCKAD), and then all three go their separate ways, with leucine to acetyl CoA and acetoacetate as the end products (as it is catabolized by only the ketogenic pathway), valine to succinyl CoA as its end product (as it is catabolized only by the glucogenic pathway), and isoleucine making succinyl CoA and acetyl CoA (as it is catabolized by both the ketogenic and glucogenic pathways). BCAT comes in two forms—BCAT1, the cytoplasmic form of the enzyme, and BCAT2, the mitochondrial form of the enzyme. However, for our purposes, both of these isoforms do the same thing, by beginning the process for catabolizing branched chain amino acids. There are other aminotransferases, and in fact all amino acids have their own aminotransferase except threonine and lysine, but the three discussed above represent the aminotransferases with the most metabolic relevance, and all have the same general process—an amino acid plus alpha-keto acid produces another amino acid and alpha-keto acid (Figure 5.3A).

> **Pancakes anyone?**
>
> A mutation in one of the subunits that makes up the BCKAD enzyme results in condition called: Maple Syrup Urine Disease. In this condition, branched chain amino acids are not fully catabolized, and rather are found in the urine, giving it a dark maple syrup like color, and a sweet smell. Hence the name.

Before we leave the topic of the aminotransferases, we should address the question you all are wondering…what happens to all of that glutamate that is made? In other words, you are probably thinking, isn't this catabolism, which would mean breaking down amino acids? Yes, that is true, but in some cases, we are using glutamate in protein synthesis (anabolism). However, more glutamate is made than is usually needed, and that is where glutamate dehydrogenase comes in (Figure 5.4A). Let's talk about deamination.

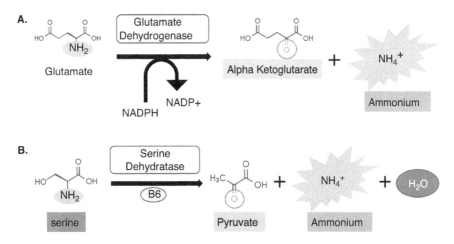

Figure 5.4: **Deaminases.** Deaminases generally remove amide groups from the side chains of amino acids, leaving an alpha-keto acid and ammonium ion. Deaminases can be either dehydrogenase enzymes such as glutamate dehydrogenase (**A**), or dehydratase enzymes such as serine dehydratase (**B**).

Deamination

Deamination simply refers to the reactions, catalyzed by dehydrogenases or dehydratases, in which the amino group is removed from a molecule. Think "de" (remove), "amin" (amino), "ation" (reaction). Dehydrogenases transfer hydrogens in an oxidation-reduction reaction, using NADPH in the case of deaminases. An example is glutamate dehydrogenase, which forms an alpha-keto acid such as alpha ketoglutarate, and an ammonium ion (Figure 5.4A). On the other hand, serine dehydratase uses vitamin B6, and forms water, along with pyruvate and an ammonium ion (Figure 5.4B). Take a look back at Figure 5.2, and what you'll see is that serine is a glucogenic amino acid, because when it is catabolized, it is converted to pyruvate, which can be shuttled into gluconeogenesis. Similarly, glutamate is also glucogenic and can be catabolized into alpha ketoglutarate, entering the TCA cycle.

Another important deaminase is glutaminase, which interconverts glutamine and glutamate (Figure 5.5A). The reaction can take place in the brain, liver hepatocytes, and in the kidney. In all of these cells, excess ammonium can be disposed of by converting glutamate and ammonium to glutamine, another amino acid[2]. In fact, glutamine is the most abundant amino acid found in blood serum. In brain, this is the preferred direction of the reaction[2]. However, the reaction catalyzed by glutaminase is reversible, and in liver, depending on needs, glutamine can be picked up from circulation and converted to glutamate and ammonium for waste disposal. Different sets of hepatocytes make a different enzyme. Glutamine synthetase (Figure 5.5B) is also highly expressed in muscle and lung cells[3]. In the brain, neurons make glutaminase, while astrocytes make glutamine synthetase. Together this is referred to as the glutamine-glutamate cycle.

There are two types of hepatocytes in the liver that work together to dispose of ammonium. The periportal hepatocytes are the first cells exposed to ammonium in circulation and can uptake the ammonium, sending it to the urea cycle (Figure 5.6). These cells also uptake glutamine and through glutaminase, release additional ammonium ions to the urea cycle. This leaves the periportal hepatocytes with glutamate left over that can be excreted. The second set of hepatocytes are called perivenous hepatocytes. The perivenous hepatocytes are the back-up system for ammonium removal. They pick up remaining ammonium that the periportal

Figure 5.5: **The Glutamine-Glutamate Cycle.** (**A**) Glutamine can be deaminated to glutamate and an ammonium ion with the addition of some water. Note that the -NH$_2$ group on glutamine is removed and changed to -OH group on glutamate. This reaction is freely reversible. In neurons, the liver, and the kidney, glutamate produced from aminotransferases is converted to glutamine, which also rids cells of ammonium. (**B**) Glutamine synthase is an alternate mechanism, which operates in astrocytes of the brain and in the liver (in separate cells from those expressing glutaminase). Glutamine synthase uses one ATP in the process, and is not reversible.

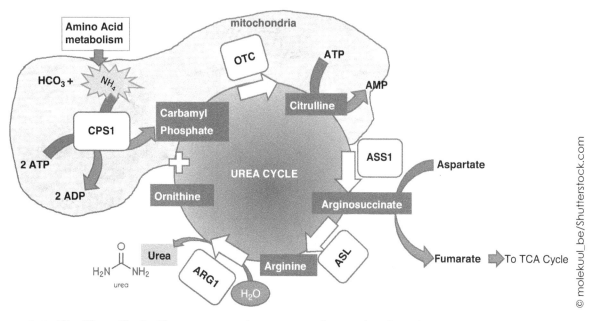

Figure 5.6: **The Urea Cycle**. Two waste products, ammonium and carbon dioxide are disposed of, making urea. Key enzymes, ornithine transcarbamylase (OTC), arginosuccinate synthetase 1 (ASS1), argininosuccinic acid lyase (ASL), arginase 1 (ARG1), and carbamoyl phosphate synthetase 1 (CPS1), are indicated in green boxes. Note that the fumarate that is produced can enter the TCA cycle, producing one NADH molecule.

hepatocytes missed and can also uptake glutamate. The perivenous hepatocytes don't have a urea cycle. Instead they use glutamine synthetase to add the ammonium ion to glutamate producing a harmless glutamine amino acid that can be released into circulation.

In general, the glutamine synthetase enzyme acts to rid cells of ammonium, making glutamine which can safely shuttle nitrogen to the liver or, if made by the liver, out into circulation for use by cells as an amino acid. The level of urea produced by the liver is determined by adjusting the need for the amino acid glutamine, against, the amino acid and neurotransmitter glutamate, in the body.

Amine-group Disposal

Once the nitrogen is removed from amino acids using aminotransferases and deaminases, the carbon skeleton of the amino acid is shuttled to either the glucogenic or ketogenic pathway, as shown in Figure 5.2. The amine group, which has been converted to ammonium, is shuttled to the urea cycle for eventual disposal in urine. As show in Figure 5.6, ammonium and HCO_3 (made from CO_2—also a waste product) can be converted to carbamoyl phosphate and added to ornithine to make citrulline in the first two steps of the urea cycle (via carbamoyl phosphate synthetase 1 and ornithine transcarbamylase) inside the mitochondria. Citrulline with the addition of an aspartate amino acid are then converted to arginosuccinate in the cytosol via arginosuccinate synthetase 1, which is broken into arginine (an amino acid) and fumarate (which can enter the TCA cycle) by argininosuccinic acid lyase. Finally, arginine is brokendown into urea and ornithine via arginase 1. The urea is released into blood to be filtered out by the kidney. The ornithine re-enters the mitochondria for continuation of the urea cycle. As the first two enzymes of the cycle, namely carbamoyl phosphate synthase, and ornithine transcarbamylase, are only expressed in liver, this really limits the urea cycle to the liver[4]. Thus, the main disposal of amine groups is through liver metabolism. Note that the initial enzyme

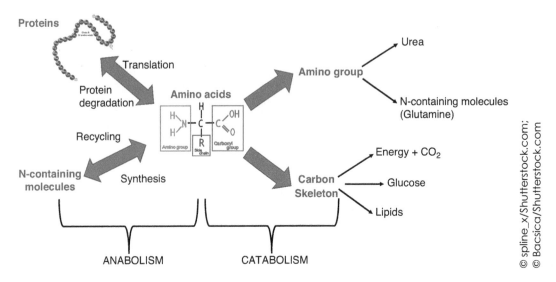

Figure 5.7: **Protein Catabolism and Anabolism.** Amino acids can be used to make proteins (translation), and proteins can be degraded to yield amino acids (proteolysis). Anabolism or synthesis of nitrogen containing molecules from amino acids, creates molecules such as carnitine or glutathione. Catabolism or degradation of amino acids breaks them into carbon skeletons for energy production, and ammonium, mostly used for urea production.

in the urea cycle requires 2 ATP molecules, while the third step uses an additional ATP, converting it to AMP, making waste disposal an energy-requiring system of the equivalent of 4 ATP. However, clean-up has to be done, and to rid itself of toxic ammonium, the body gladly donates the energy. In addition, since fumarate is produced, one NADH molecule can be made in the TCA cycle upon its entry, and this negates the ATP use by generating 2.5 ATPs back. Don't you love how the body is so good at recycling?

Summary

Twenty amino acids are genetically encoded by mRNAs, attached to tRNAs, and together these produce proteins. We have the ability to produce a vast array of protein simply by putting together different combinations of amino acids in the protein chain. Thus, as each amino acid has its own unique characteristics in terms of charge, hydrophobicity, acidity or basic properties, and other side chains (such as those with sulfur or aromatic rings), that can uniquely specify function, place it in specific sites the cell or extracellular spaces, and influence 3D folding.

Important to amino acid metabolism, is the concept of amino acid synthesis and catabolism (Figure 5.7). Humans can only synthesize a few amino acids *de novo* and can make some others from spare parts. The rest are essential, meaning that to use those amino acids, we must ingest them first. In addition, once we are done with a protein and it is broken down into individual amino acids, we will either recycle those amino acids into new proteins or turn them into ammonium. As ammonium is quite toxic to the body, it is removed either through the production of glutamine, which safely transports nitrogen/amide groups in its side chain, or through urea production and urination.

Points to Ponder

➤ What determines whether an amino acid undergoes glucogenic, ketogenic, or both types of catabolism? Is there any easy way that you can come up with to remember the designations?

➤ Why have two cell types in brain and liver—one that makes glutamine synthase and the other that makes glutaminase? Is there a metabolic purpose for the glutamine-glutamate cycle?

➤ Since glutamine synthase requires one ATP, but glutamate dehydrogenase takes an NADPH, wouldn't it be more energy efficient for the body to simply dispose of all glutamate through glutamine synthase? Why or why not?

References

1. Wolfe RR. Branched-chain amino acids and muscle protein synthesis in humans: myth or reality? *J Int Soc Sports Nutr.* 2017;14:30.
2. Yudkoff M. Interactions in the Metabolism of Glutamate and the Branched-Chain Amino Acids and Ketoacids in the CNS. *Neurochem Res.* 2017;42(1):10–18.
3. Meynial-Denis D. Glutamine metabolism in advanced age. *Nutr Rev.* 2016;74(4):225–236.
4. Summar ML, Mew NA. Inborn Errors of Metabolism with Hyperammonemia: Urea Cycle Defects and Related Disorders. *Pediatr Clin North Am.* 2018;65(2):231–246.

The Fed State

CHAPTER 6

Let's eat and digest

Once we eat a meal, no matter what it was, the postprandial period (or the period of time following the meal) is the time during which the meal is digested by various parts of our digestive system where it can be absorbed, the nutrient components of the meal (macronutrients, i.e., carbohydrates, proteins, and fat) are transported, and within specific tissues, the macronutrients are metabolized. This entire process takes about 4–6 hours to complete (so if you eat breakfast at 8 AM, by the time the noon, lunchtime, you might still be digesting breakfast!). As we will see, meals with lots of fats and proteins take longer to digest than high carbohydrate meals. Each type of macronutrient has its own specialized enzymes and absorption mechanisms. In this chapter, each will be discussed in detail.

Digestion and Absorption

Let's look at the individual steps of digestion of food as a whole (Figure 6.1). In the mouth, food is masticated (a fancy word meaning it is chewed), and moistened with saliva, which contains some enzymes for simple breakdown of food. Think about how hard it would be to swallow a saltine cracker without saliva and you'll realize its importance. The tongue not only has taste buds to help us enjoy the food (and recognize food versus poison), but also is a strong group of muscles, which can push the food around in our mouth, and help correctly position it for swallowing. Food is then transported through the esophagus, aided by peristaltic contractions of the smooth muscles surrounding the esophagus. The esophagus has sphincters at its top and bottom. You might think these are under voluntary control, or at least that the upper one is, but it's not. The upper esophageal sphincter is opened following the swallowing reflex, while the lower esophageal sphincter is completely under the control of autonomic (involuntary) nerves. Once the food empties into the stomach, a slurry of mucous and acid in the stomach as well as enzymes from the gastric cells, further break down the chunks of food coming from the mouth. This is where digestion really gets going! The stomach has to create a mass of mush (called chyme—which is a liquefied slurry food mix) and creates a great environment for food digestion

> **Did you know?**
>
> The average human stomach can hold about 1 liter of food, and our entire digestive system can handle about 9 liters of food and water per day.

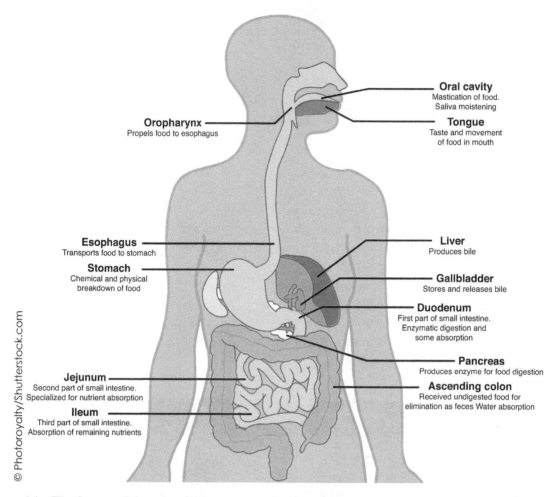

© Photoroyalty/Shutterstock.com

Figure 6.1: **The human Digestive System.** Parts and function of the human digestive system are shown.

in the small intestine. The stomach also can do some absorption—of water, some medications, alcohol, and some vitamins. However, most of the chyme gets pushed into the small intestine after somewhere between forty minutes to several hours (depending on the macronutrient content of the food). Only a little bit of chyme at a time enters the duodenum, which is the first section (and the shortest section) of the small intestine. Proteins, fats, and carbohydrates are further broken down by intestinal enzymes, and also absorbed here as the food moves through the duodenum, jejunum, and ileum before leaving for the large intestine, where water and some nutrients (i.e. certain vitamins and short-chained fatty acids) are absorbed before the formation of feces and elimination of waste. With that introduction to the process, let's get into the details of the upper digestive track, including the mouth and stomach as well as talk about the role of the small intestine in digestion of macronutrients.

Carbohydrate Digestion and Absorption

Carbohydrates—both the simple and complex carbohydrates start digestion in the mouth. Take a look back at Figure 3.1 to remind yourself about the different categories of carbohydrates. Three salivary glands in the mouth work to start the digestion process—the paired parotid glands which are found on either side of the mouth, the submandibular glands, and the smallest ones— the sublingual glands (Figure 6.2A). These glands produce saliva, as well as a mucous fluid which can both work to lubricate and moisten food, and aid in mastication. Only the parotid and submandibular glands produce the salivary gland enzyme "salivary gland alpha amylase". This enzyme is a glycosidase that hydrolyses the alpha-1,4 glyosidic bonds of polysaccharides (Figure 6.2B, C). However, the beta-1,4 bonds which are found in cellulose and lactose, as well as the alpha 1,6 branch points of amylopectin are resistant to digestion by this enzyme. What this enzyme can do is to cleave larger polysaccharides such as starch (amylose and amylopectin) and glycogen (only exists in trace amounts in the diet), producing dextrins (short branched polysaccharides), oligosaccharides, and some mono- or disaccharides, including glucose, maltose, and sucrose. This starts the carbohydrate digestion process. Interestingly, dogs, and wolves—obligate carnivores that would have very low ingestion of starches do not make salivary amylase at all—only pancreatic amylase which we will talk more about shortly. Humans, and other animals, such as mice make both salivary and pancreatic amylase[2]. As the digested mono-, di-, and polysaccharides move in the stomach, there is now no further breakdown of carbohydrates because the acidic environment of the stomach (from HCl released by the parietal cells) inhibits the activity of salivary alpha-amylase.

> **Chew slowly...**
>
> The longer you chew, the more thoroughly sugars and fats can be broken down by salivary amylase and lingual lipase. If you swallow quickly without chewing thoroughly, these enzymes won't have a lot of time to work, and you won't taste your food as well.

> **Interesting genetic fact**
>
> Humans have anywhere between 2 to 17 copies (duplications) of the AMY1 gene which codes for amylase. The variation in number of copies appears to be related to ethnicity, with populations who eat a lot starch (i.e. Japanese and Europeans) having more copies than individuals from populations that traditionally eat less starch (i.e. Biaka of central Africa)[1].

As the chyme containing carbohydrates move into the small intestine (SI), they encounter a more neutral environment, due to high bicarbonate levels, which help to neutralize the pH of the slurry

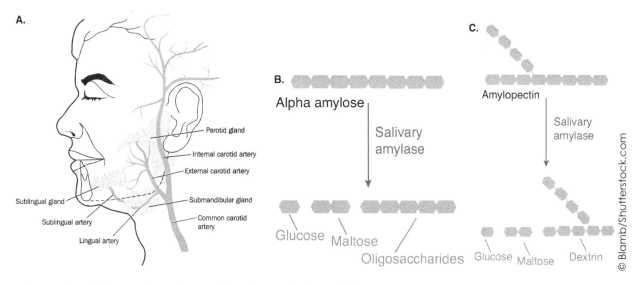

Figure 6.2: **Salivary Glands and Starches. (A)** Three different paired salivary glands secrete salivary enzymes and saliva to moisten foods and begin breaking down starch and other carbohydrates. Salivary amylase can cleave both forms of starch, alpha amylose **(B)** and amylopectin **(C)** by cleaving the α1-4 glycosidic bonds. Note that the branched β1-4, α1-2, and α1-6 glycosidic bonds are resistant to cleavage.

coming from the stomach. As the chyme enters the SI, it triggers enteroendocrine cells to release their hormones: cholecystokinin (CCK) and secretin, which travel to the pancreas. Secretin stimulates the pancreatic acinar cells to release bicarbonate and CCK stimulates the acinar cells to release pancreatic enzymes. Bicarbonate and pancreatic enzymes travel down the pancreatic duct, joining with the bile duct, which empties into the duodenum. Bicarbonate raises the pH and helps the carbohydrate-digesting enzymes to maintain their enzymatic activity and breakdown carbohydrates to glucose, galactose, and fructose. The brush border of the small intestine, with all of its microvilli and large surface area can absorb at least 5400 g/day of glucose and 54.7 g/day of fructose. Consider how much glucose and fructose (especially those foods with hidden high fructose corn syrup in them) you consume in a day—can you absorb it all? Most likely, yes but that is still a lot of simple carbohydrates.

Before we get to that, let's talk a little more about the small intestine and these enzymes, which are coming from the pancreas and intestinal enterocytes (which are SI absorptive cells that produce brush border enzymes). Pancreatic juices are secreted into the small intestine at a rate of about 1.2–1.5 liters be day. The pancreatic juice is a combination of water, bicarbonate for stom-

> **It's a fact!**
> Vampire bats are the only known vertebrate not to secrete the intestinal maltase enzyme.

ach acid neutralization, and enzymes for digesting carbohydrates, proteins, and lipids. For now, let's focus on the major pancreatic enzyme that targets carbohydrates—pancreatic alpha-amylase. Just like salivary alpha-amylase, pancreatic amylase does not need to be activated—it is ready to work on digestion straight-away[3]. No other pancreatic enzymes are needed for starch and simple carbohydrate digestion in the small intestine—rather intestinal enterocytes produce several carbohydrate-specific enzymes to further break down the carbohydrates to glucose, galactose, and fructose. These are further described on Table 6.1. The brush border enzymes: maltase, sucrase, isomaltase, and lactase cleave their target disaccharides to produce glucose, galactose, and fructose. Glucose, galactose, and fructose can be absorbed for transport and energy production by other cells in the body.

Table 6.1: **Intestinal carbohydrate-targeting enzymes**.

Enzyme	Target	Products	Other Info
Pancreatic Alpha amylase	Starch	Glucose, maltose, dextrins	• Cleaves the α1-4 bond of starch • Secreted by pancreatic acinar cells
Maltase	Maltose and maltotriose	Glucose	• Cleaves the α1-4 bond of dextrins • Made by enterocytes & inserted on the brush border
Sucrase	Sucrose	Fructose and glucose	• Cleaves the α1-2 bond of sucrose • Made by enterocytes & inserted on the brush border
Isomaltase	Dextrins	Glucose	• Cleaves the α1-6 bond of dextrins • Made by enterocytes & inserted on the brush border
Lactase	Lactose	Glucose and galactose	• Cleaves the β1-4 bond between galactose and glucose • Made by enterocytes & inserted on the brush border • Activity decreases in some people with age, leading to lactose intolerance

Once digested into monosaccharides, glucose and other simple carbohydrates (grouped together with the name "hexose," a 6-carbon carbohydrate or "pentose," a 5-carbon carbohydrate) must get absorbed. However, this is not as simple as just diffusing in. Monosaccharide transporters are found on the apical (or luminal) membrane side of the enterocyte, which is the side of the cell that faces into the lumen of the small intestine. The other side of the cell, termed the basolateral membrane, is key for transport of the absorbed molecules into the bloodstream (Figure 6.3). The small intestinal wall itself is very folded and convoluted. As shown on Figure 6.3, the lining of the small intestine is first folded into circular folds. On each fold are finger-like projections called villi, which themselves are made up of individual enterocyte cells with microvilli, or small hair-like structures on their luminal side. This folding allows for significantly increased surface area—in other words, more places to absorb nutrients.

Different types of sugars use different transporters. Both glucose and galactose use the **s**odium **glu**cose **t**ransporter-**1** (SGLT1) which co-transports one glucose molecule or one galactose molecule with two sodium (Na^+) ions (Figure 6.4). Note that sodium levels in the enterocyte must also be maintained, so a Na^+/K^+ pump is used to pump three Na^+ ions back out, while bringing in two K^+ ions, to maintain cellular water and ion homeostasis. The Na^+/K^+ pump, sometimes referred to as a Na^+/K^+ ATPase, requires ATP, therefore this type of transport is called secondary active transport. ATP is used

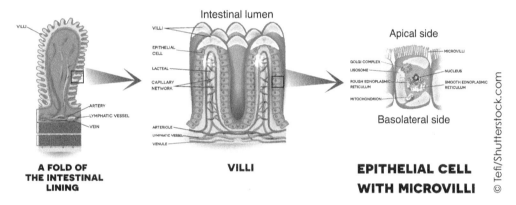

Figure 6.3: **Small Intestinal Villi.** The intestinal lumen is highly folded with each circular fold having many villi. Each villi is then composed of many cells (specifically enterocytes), each having lots of microvilli on them.

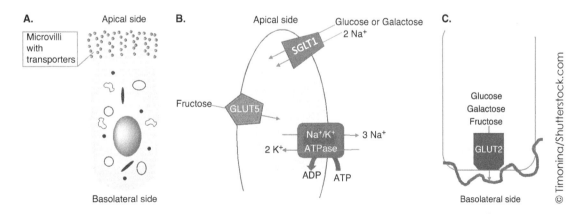

Figure 6.4: **Glucose, Galactose, and Fructose Absorption by Small Intestine Enterocytes. (A)** An enterocyte with microvilli. Each microvilli has many different transporters for absorption. **(B)** Close up of a microvillus with SGLT1, GLUT5, and the Na^+/K^+ ATPase. **(C)** Close up of basolateral side of enterocyte with GLUT2. Glucose, galactose, and fructose are are transported directly into the microcapillary bed by facilitated diffusion.

secondarily through the Na^+/K^+ pump, but not directly with SGLT1. Fructose on the other hand does not require Na^+ ions or ATP—rather it can be absorbed using the GLUT5 transporter (Figure 6.4), which uses facilitated diffusion for transport. Facilitated diffusion involves transport along a concentration gradient (which means going from areas with high levels of the diffused substance to areas of low concentrations). In this case, the GLUT5 transporter recognizes fructose molecules among the slurry of other things in the small intestine and *facilitates* its diffusion across the apical membrane of the enterocyte. All of the monosaccharides that we just discussed get transported into the enterocyte, and then need to get out to the bloodstream (unless the enterocyte uses them). Transport at the basolateral membrane occurs through the GLUT2 transporter (Figure 6.4). This transporter also uses facilitated diffusion, again taking advantage of concentration gradients to transport glucose, galactose, and fructose to the extracellular fluids, including the blood. The capillaries that feed the SI drain into the portal vein of the liver and then are transported to other cells in the body. We'll talk about where these monosaccharides are used later, but not within this section of the textbook.

Transport and Distribution of Carbohydrates

As we finish a meal, the primary objective of the body is to digest, distribute, and store the macronutrients. This is considered to be an *anabolic* period—a period of storage and building, rather than energy generation (*catabolic*). In this period of transport and distribution, carbohydrate absorption stimulates insulin secretion, and insulin is our key hormone in this process. Insulin is produced and released from the beta cells of the pancreas. As we will see in this section (and in later chapters describing transport and distribution of digested lipids and proteins/amino acids), insulin stimulates glucose uptake and storage; ATP synthesis from glucose; lipid uptake, storage, and new lipid synthesis; and protein synthesis, that will ultimately determine whether energy is stored or used.

Glucose Transport and Clearance

Pancreatic beta cells have a glucose transporter, GLUT2, which has a high Km—or high ability to transport glucose with increasing concentrations of glucose in the blood serum after a meal. Thus there is an increased uptake of glucose into the beta cells with food intake. As glucose enters the beta cell, it is immediately phosphorylated by glucokinase (found in the liver and pancreas), forming glucose-6-phosphate (Figure 6.5A). The enzyme glucokinase is also a high Km enzyme—which means that when a high concentration of glucose is sensed inside the beta cells, glucokinase activity is stimulated, resulting in phosphorylation of glucose and production of glucose-6-phosphate. The concentration must be very high (i.e. around 5 mM, the physiological range, or above) to get glucose phosphorylation[4]. Take a look at Figure 6.5B to see how concentration of glucose affects glucokinase activity compared to hexokinase in skeletal muscle. Based on the different energy needs and roles of many types of cells and organs in the body, it is important (described in more detail below) that glucose metabolism is regulated differently in the beta cells of the pancreas compared to other cell types. Glucose-6-phosphate then enters glycolysis, forming pyruvate which eventually forms ATP through oxidative phosphorylation. This series of events in which the rise in substrate, namely glucose, results in increased ATP levels, blocks ATP-sensitive potassium channels, blocking potassium efflux (release). This depolarizes the cell, due to changes in potassium concentrations within the cell $[K^+]$ resulting in activation of voltage-gated calcium channels. These voltage-gated calcium channels open allowing an influx of calcium into the cell. Calcium facilitates the docking and exocytosis of insulin containing vesicles, releasing insulin from the beta cell. This makes sense, because only when glucose levels are high (hence the higher Km mentioned above) will we have a threshold high enough to release insulin from the beta cell—and this means that in fasted individuals, insulin won't be released, and glucose homeostasis is maintained.

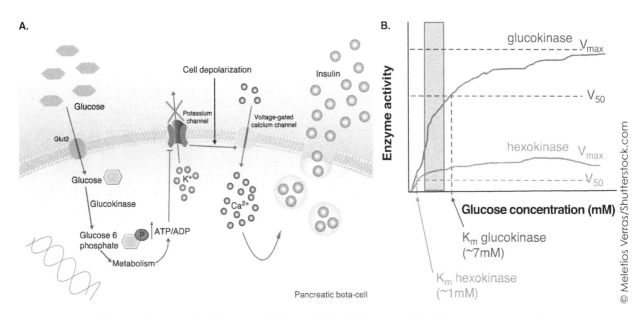

Figure 6.5: **Glucose Sensing by Pancreatic Beta Cells. (A)** Beta cells within pancreatic islets have GLUT2 transporters. Upon uptake, insulin is released from intercellular vesicles through a series of steps including glucokinase phosphorylation, glycolysis and TCA cycle generation of ATP, voltage-gated channel blockage of the release of potassium, membrane depolarization, calcium influx, and release of insulin from secretory granules. **(B)** Glucokinase enzymatic activity is dependent on glucose concentration on the cell, with higher levels of glucose needed to stimulate high activity of the enzyme than with hexokinase. Approximate fasting blood glucose ranges shown by red bar.

Think about other cells—do you think their glucose receptors and glucokinase enzymes would have a high or a low Km? In other words, when there is glucose around, how do they respond? For example, in an alpha cell which produces glucagon, or a brain cell that needs the glucose for energy metabolism, the Kms of both of these cellular transporters is much lower. More about this later!

Insulin release from the beta cell results in a lot of systemic activity. For example, insulin triggers uptake of free fatty acids, glucose, and amino acids. It triggers glycogen production and inhibits glycogen breakdown (catabolic pathway). Insulin also inhibits triglyceride breakdown and gluco-neogenesis in the liver. In general insulin stimulates anabolic pathways—or those that promote uptake and storage of macronutrients. However, one catabolic pathway is still active—glycolysis. With the high levels of circulating glucose, glycolysis is favored for ATP production over fatty acid metabolism.

As insulin circulates in the blood stream, cells with insulin receptors will bind insulin (Figure 6.6A, B). This causes a cascade of events in the cells, resulting in phosphorylation of the insulin receptor as well as a number of other signaling proteins such as the IRS1, IRS2, IRS3, and IRS4 kinases, and the Gab-1 kinases. As we'll see, glucose transporters are translocated to the cell surface, resulting in glucose uptake by the cell.

Glucose Transporters

There are 14 known glucose transporters, and most, except for GLUT4 are **not** regulated by insulin (Table 6.2)[5]. In other words, for most of these, like we just saw with GLUT2 in pancreatic beta cells, there is NOT an insulin-dependent uptake of glucose. But for GLUT4, which is expressed mainly in striated muscle (skeletal muscle) and adipose tissue, insulin stimulation causes uptake of glucose by

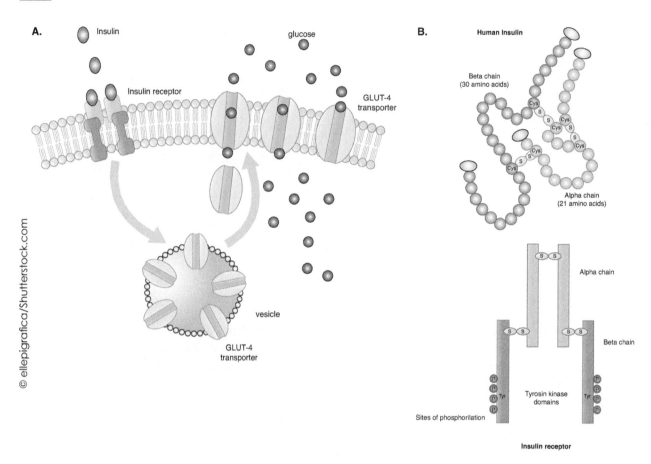

© ellepigrafica/Shutterstock.com

Figure 6.6: **Insulin Signaling and GLUT4 Translocation.** (**A**) Insulin binds to cellular insulin receptor which causes GLUT4 translocation to the plasma membrane surface. (**B**) Amino acid structure of human insulin, and the insulin receptor.

Table 6.2: **Main glucose transporters.**

Glucose Transporter	Insulin Response	K_m mM, substrate	Expression
GLUT1	No	5 mM, glucose	Erythrocytes, blood brain barrier, fetal tissues
GLUT2	No	10–15 mM, glucose, galactose, fructose	Liver, beta cells of pancreas, kidney, intestine
GLUT3	No	1–2 mM, glucose	Neurons
GLUT4	Yes	3-5 mM, glucose	Skeletal muscle, heart, brown and white adipocytes
GLUT5	No	6 mM, fructose	Intestine, testis, kidney

translocating GLUT4 to the cell membrane. High circulating levels of glucose (hyperglycemia) can damage small capillaries and therefore, glucose needs to be removed from the serum—and striated muscle and adipose tissue are the tissues able to do this. In fact, skeletal muscle can take up 60–80% of circulating glucose in the presence of insulin. GLUT4 has a K_m that corresponds to normal physiological levels of glucose (3.5—5.5 mM), which means in the presence of both insulin and high glucose concentrations, skeletal muscle quickly disposes of circulating glucose. On the other hand, GLUT3, which is mainly expressed in the brain has a low Km, meaning that even in low serum glucose levels (i.e. you are just waking up in the morning after not eating since dinner the night before), glucose will be taken in by brain cells. This is also really important—the brain, and in particular many neurons, rely on glucose at the primary source of energy, so they must be able to grab the available glucose in serum, no matter how low that level goes. Brain will get the glucose before tissues like muscle or adipose tissue, for example.

So, how does GLUT4 grab the glucose in striated muscle and adipose tissues? In the resting state, only 3–10% of GLUT4 transporters are on the membrane while the rest of the GLUT4 proteins are in intracellular storage vesicles within the cytoplasm of the cell (Figure 6.6A). As insulin binds to insulin receptors on the cell membrane, an intracellular signaling cascade results in GLUT4 transporters being released by these vesicles as they move to the cell membrane of the cell and fuse with it. This results in the ability of the cell (striated muscle or adipose tissue) to take up even more glucose[6,7].

All of these processes are focused on the clearance of glucose from circulation with high blood glucose levels by stimulating glucose uptake in the beta cell and subsequent insulin release, and then stimulation of insulin-sensitive cells (such as striated muscle and adipose tissue) to take up even more glucose. In addition, the liver is also taking up glucose and forming glycogen for later use. All of these pathways lead to clearance of glucose from circulation, usage of glucose for ATP synthesis, and the storage of glucose for later use by skeletal muscle and liver.

Other Monosaccharides

While high glucose levels stimulate insulin release from the pancreas, this is not the case for galactose and fructose, where their metabolism in the liver. Cellular uptake of fructose and galactose by GLUT2 in the liver requires facilitated transport. Galactose can then be converted to glucose-6-phosphate, by several enzymatic steps (galactolysis) and either enter glycolysis or be stored as glycogen. Fructose on the other hand, has a longer metabolic pathway (fructolysis) resulting in the glycolysis intermediate: glyceraldehyde-3-phosphate. From there, the glyceraldehyde-3-phosphate can finish glycolysis, be used to form glucose (gluconeogenesis), or be converted to glycerol-3-phosphate, the backbone of triglycerides. The liver is the primary metabolizer of galactose and fructose, since other tissues don't really need or use them, and really rely almost solely on glucose for their energy needs. In fact, we generally say that glucose is the most nutritionally important monosaccharide.

Fat Absorption, Transport and Clearance

Digestion and Absorption

The mouth is also the place where we start to digest lipids. It turns out that in addition to the main salivary glands, we also have what are termed "minor" salivary glands which are non-encapsulated, but present within the connective tissue or around and within the muscle fibers of the tongue[8]. Many of these minor glands secrete mucous, an important part of the saliva, which is needed for moisturizing and emulsifying lipids. Both the major and minor salivary glands secrete lipids into the saliva, and these are thought to help with transport and uptake of digested lipids through the oral cavity[9]. However, before absorption of ingested lipids,

> **Fun Fact**
> Pancreatic lipase is not produced in infants, as they do not have a fully formed pancreas. Thus, breast milk is full of free fatty acids, rather than TAGs to help in infant digestion. However, more recent work has shown that a second protein, called pancreatic lipase-related protein-2 (PLRP2) is secreted by infants and can work to digest mono-, di- and triglycerides[10].

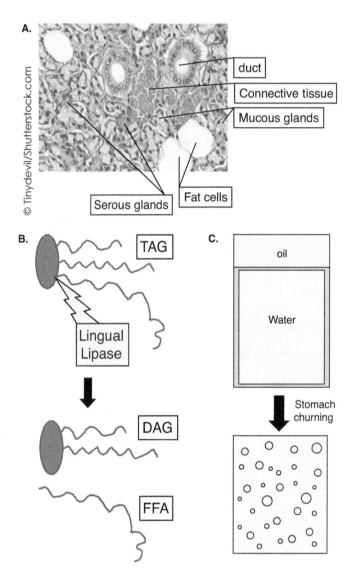

Figure 6.7: **Lipid Digestion in the Mouth and Stomach.** (**A**) Histological view of a minor salivary gland. Note the connective tissue, serous glands secreting proteins, and mucous glands secreting salivary mucous. (**B**) Cartoon of a triglyceride with different length fatty acids. Lingual Lipase (as well as gastric lipase) preferentially cleave the third carbon of a triglyceride (TAG), forming a diglyceride (DAG), and a free fatty acid (FFA). (**C**) Within the stomach, lipids are emulsified by the stomach's constant churning into droplets that can enter the small intestine.

digestion must take place. The enzyme lingual lipase, which is secreted from a minor salivary serous gland behind the tongue, starts the digestion process (Figure 6.7A). This enzyme is responsible for cleaving the ester bond at the number 3 carbon on some triglycerides forming a free fatty acid and 1,2-diglyceride (Figure 6.7B). Lingual lipase has optimal enzymatic activity at a pH of 4.0, which means as the dietary lipids travel to the stomach, both lingual lipase, and gastric lipase which is produced by the stomach, work to digest fats in the stomach. As these lipases preferentially work on short and medium-chain triglycerides, only about 10–30% of the fats in the stomach are digested at this point. The other important process going on in the stomach is emulsification (Figure 6.7C), where fats are mixed with the hydrophilic juices of the stomach by peristaltic movements of the smooth muscles surrounding the stomach, allowing for enzymes to gain access to the TAGs for

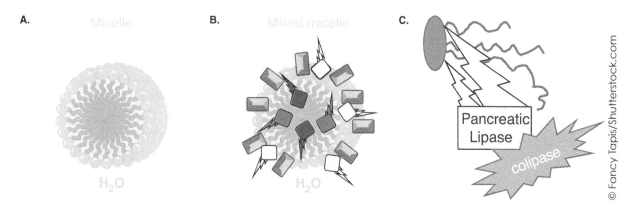

Figure 6.8: **Lipid Digestion within the Small Intestine.** (A) Micelles have hydrophilic heads and hydrophobic tails composed of phospholipids and form themselves into a sphere containing lipids and lipid-digesting enzymes inside. These form in the stomach and enter the small intestine, where they come in contact with enzymes and bile salts. (B) Bile salts coat the micelle and enzymes are packaged within the micelle, forming a mixed micelle. However, while most enzymes are active at this stage, pancreatic lipase (in yellow) is not. (C) With the action of colipase, pancreatic lipase gains access to lipids and can cleave the first or third carbon off of the glycerol on a triglyceride, forming a diglyceride or monoglyceride, and free fatty acids.

digestion due to the increased surface area of individual droplets, compared to large layers of fat that might have been present when the meal was initially dropped into the stomach. Un-emulsified lipids can delay stomach emptying, such that until the lipid droplets are fully emulsified, they simply do not leave for the small intestine. This is one of the reasons that a higher fat meal can result in a feeling of fullness for longer than might occur with a high carbohydrate meal.

As the lipids enter the small intestine, the real work in digesting lipids occur here as 95% of all dietary fat ingested is absorbed[10]. As mentioned earlier, pancreatic juices emptying into the small intestine are full of bicarbonate, which can neutralize the acidic chyme coming from the stomach. CCK, the enzyme that causes pancreatic enzymes to be released, also works on the gall bladder to release bile. Bile salts then empty into the small intestine, allowing for even more emulsification of the emptying stomach contents, and together all of this allows for more cleavage of lipid molecules and release of free fatty acids by enzymes. Phospholipids from the diet combine to produce micelles (Figure 6.8A). Micelles are single-layer lipid bubbles that have a hydrophilic outside with a hydrophobic inside. Within micelles, the free fatty acids, cholesterol, fat-soluble vitamins, triglycerides, and other lipid breakdown products are packaged into a little compartment, which, along with co-packaged enzymes such as phospholipase A_2 and cholesterol esterase that continue to break down the lipids. These are then mixed with bile salts coming from the gallbladder to form mixed micelles (Figure 6.8B). Phospholipase A_2 works on phospholipids, cleaving one of the two fatty acids, which produces a free fatty acid and lysophosphatidylcholine. Cholesterol esterase works on cholesterol esters (a cholesterol with a fatty acid attached) to produce a free fatty acid and cholesterol.

In the SI, pancreatic juice enters and contains pancreatic lipase, as well as a second protein, pancreatic lipase related protein 2 (PLRP2), which can both interact with the mixed micelle, but pancreatic lipase then requires a second pancreatic protein, colipase, to become fully active. PLRP2 on the other hand is active without colipase, but can use colipase to become even more active[10]. Together, these enzymes work to cleave the remaining triglycerides at carbon 1 and carbon 3 into 2-monoglycerides (MAGs) and free fatty acids (Figure 6.8C), which are packed together within the mixed micelle.

Depending on the concentration of fats in the small intestine, two different systems can then be used for uptake of fats into enterocytes. If concentrations of fats are high, then micelles are simply fused with the enterocyte membrane and the contents dumped into the cell. If concentrations are low, then facilitated diffusion, using a fatty acid transporter FATP4 or FAT/CD36, can be used to pick up fatty acids and other lipids from the intestinal slurry and transport them into the enterocyte. Once inside the enterocyte, the lipids are resynthesized into their pre-digestion form. The MAGs pick up two fatty acids becoming a TAG again, cholesterol picks up

> **Did you know?**
>
> Individuals with a genetic variant affecting their ability to synthesize ApoB (B48 and B100) proteins, have abetalipoproteinemia, which results in an inability to make mature chylomicrons. This condition affects not only lipids, but fat-soluble vitamin uptake.

one fatty acid becoming a cholesterol ester again, and lysophosphatidylcholine picks up one fatty acid becoming the phospholipid, phosphatidylcholine again. The cholesterol esters, TAGs, phospholipids, and other lipids (such as fat-soluble vitamins) are incorporated into chylomicrons within the endoplasmic reticulum and golgi apparatus. This is an important step for the distribution of lipids to efficiently travel through the bloodstream, since lipids are not water soluble. In addition to the lipids, about 2% of the chylomicrons are composed of a group of proteins called apolipoproteins. One of the most prominent apolipoproteins is B48 (apo-B48) which can be used as a measure of chylomicrons circulating in blood (Figure 6.9). Take a look back at Figure 4.8, which shows the structure and composition of chylomicrons and other lipoproteins in the body to review the composition of these particles. Nascent chylomicrons form from the small intestine, and contain just triglycerides, phospholipids, fat-soluble vitamins, cholesterol, and apo-B48 and apo-A. Chylomicrons are too big to enter into intestinal capillaries, so they enter the lymphatic system, and eventually get to the blood, where the nascent chylomicron picks up apolipoprotein C-II and E (apo C-II, apo-E) (Figure 6.9). Within capillaries, endothelial cells anchor lipoprotein lipase (LPL) (made by adipocytes and cardiac myocytes),

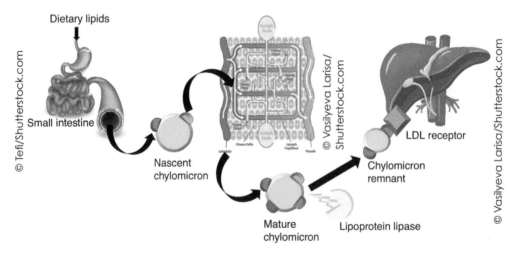

Figure 6.9: **Lipid Transport.** Dietary lipids enter the small intestine, and are released into lymph as nascent chylomicrons (yellow) with apolipoprotein B-48 (blue) and apolipoprotein A (green) on it's surface. As it enters the blood at the thoracic duct, the chylomicron picks up apolipoprotein C-II (red) and apolipoprotein E (orange). As the triglycerides in the chylomicron are hydrolyzed using lipoprotein lipase, apolipoprotein A and C-II fall off, and the chylomicron remnant is picked up by the LDL receptors, which bind to apolipoprotein E, on the liver for recycling.

which recognizes and binds to apo C-II and attacks chylomicron triglycerides[11]. Fatty acids are released and taken up by adipose tissue, and to a lesser extent skeletal muscle and other cells in the body with mitochondria, resynthesized into TAGs and stored for later use. As the mature chylomicron shrinks, and apo C-II and apo-A fall off and the now the chylomicron remnant is picked up by the liver through binding of apolipoprotein E to the liver LDL receptors (Figure 6.9). Note that chylomicrons are the predominant lipoprotein in circulation during the fed state.

After a fat-rich meal, other lipoproteins—HDLs, VLDLs, and LDLs are reduced post-prandially[12]. As the post-absorptive period begins, HDLs and VLDLs increase in circulation. The liver repackages cholesterol and TAGs into VLDLs, which are metabolized further through the action of lecithin-cholesterol acyltransferase (LCAT), and LPL, respectively (Figure 6.10). LPL again hydrolyzes VLDL triglycerides releasing free fatty acids to be taken-up by adipose tissue for storage. As the TAG content of the VLDLs decrease, they form intermediate density lipoproteins (IDL) or VLDL remnants. Note that each VLDL particle contains just one apolipoprotein B-100 (apo B-100) protein, which is absolutely required for VLDL formation[13] . Thus, availability of apo B-100 determines VLDL

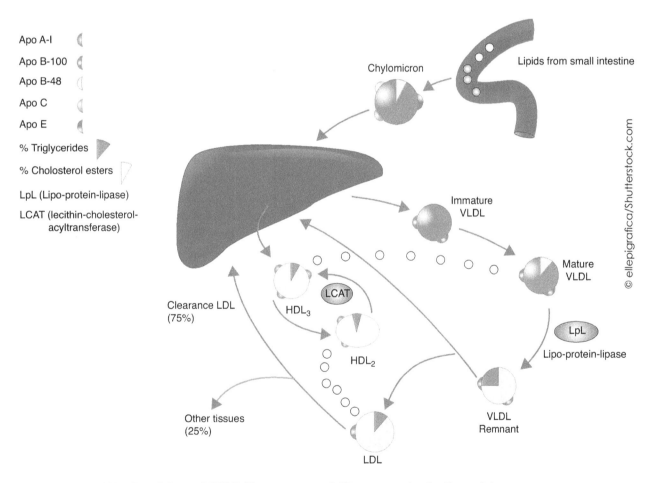

Figure 6.10: **VLDL, LDL, and HDL Transport and Clearance.** As the liver picks up nascent chylomicrons, containing ApoE, ApoB-48, and small amounts of ApoC-II, these are recycled to VLDL and HDL particles, which are released into circulation. Lipoprotein lipase further interacts with VLDL releasing TAGs, creating VLDL remnants, which eventually form LDL molecules. Lecithin-cholesterol acyltransferase (LCAT) mediates cholesterol conversion between HDL_3 and HDL_2. Fatty acids released by lipoprotein lipase can enter other lipoprotein particles or be picked up by tissues: skeletal muscle, heart, and adipose tissues.

synthesis[13]. Of the VLDL's synthesized, about 50% of these are picked up by the liver for disposal, as remnant VLDL particles. The other 50% lose ApoE, and gain cholesterol, becoming LDL particles (Figure 6.10). This is why LDL is considered the "bad" cholesterol—because LDL particles distribute cholesterol throughout the body to cells expressing an LDL receptor. High circulating LDL levels, have a well-documented associated with heath disease[14]. This is where HDL comes in…as more LDLs float around in our bloodstream, the HDL particles are also traveling the bloodstream, scavenging cholesterol from cells, and remodeling that cholesterol to cholesterol esters by LCAT[15]. This converts HDL_2 to HDL_3, and requires use another apolipoprotein, apo-A1 as an activator of the process[15] (Figure 6.10). HDL is considered the "good" cholesterol because it then can be picked up by liver HDL receptors, carrying excess cholesterol to the liver for disposal.

Fat Transport and Clearance

Free fatty acids are the only lipids that circulate in the blood and must be bound to albumin. This albumin-fatty acid complex is primarily made in adipose tissue. The rest of the lipids that we take in during a meal are incorporated into lipoproteins, primarily chylomicrons, and eventually in the post-absorptive period to a lesser extent, very low-density lipoproteins (VLDL), low density lipoproteins (LDL), and high-density lipoproteins (HDL). Generally, a lipoprotein is composed of lipid layer, with cholesterol, and apoproteins embedded in the membrane, as well as a core composed of lipids—

> **Consider these facts…**
>
> CD36 interacts with both lipids, and thrombospondin, which is involved in clotting. Some believe that these two interactions may form the basis for the role of abnormal CD36 levels (either high or low) and atherosclerosis[16]. What do you think?

cholesterol, triglycerides, fat-soluble vitamins, and free fatty acids that are being transported. Of all of the lipoproteins, the type is very dependent on whether the individual is fed or fasted. Chylomicrons are going to predominate after a meal, as these are made in the intestine, and used to transport the absorbed lipids. Chylomicrons will be reduced when we are fasted and are by far the largest in size when compared to all other lipoproteins. As the meal is digested, other types such as VLDLs, LDLs, and HDLs, which are made in the liver will rise. Interestingly, the size of the particle is inverse to the density of the particle. What we mean here is that a VLDL is larger than an LDL, but less dense. The HDL lipoprotein is the smallest and has the highest density.

As other tissues will need to pick up fatty acids for their own metabolism, specialized receptors exist to facilitate uptake. The first one we will discuss is CD36 (also called FAT…which stands for "fatty acid translocase" which is a pretty cleaver acronym, right?). FAT/CD36 interacts with many different things, including collagen, thrombospondin (a platelet protein involved in clotting), red blood cells infected with the malaria parasite, as well as LDL, oxidized LDL, and long chain fatty acids[16]. That's really a lot of interactions for a single membrane-bound receptor. For the purpose of this text, we will focus on its role in fatty acids and LDL binding. In neurons, and taste buds, expression of FAT/CD36 is linked to fatty acid sensing, while in skeletal and cardiac muscles, insulin-stimulated translocation of FAT/CD36 picks up long chain fatty acids for use in beta-oxidation[16,17]. Within cells that express FAT/CD36, this protein transporter is also present on the mitochondrial membrane, helping to transport fatty acids into the mitochondria for metabolism. Fatty acids bind to the outside area of FAT/CD36, and are transported through a tunnel within the protein made up of beta-sheets formed into columns[18] (Figure 6.11).

Fatty acid binding proteins (FABPs) are part of a family of proteins with a heme core that interact with fatty acids. FABP1 was the first family member identified, and probably is the best studied, as

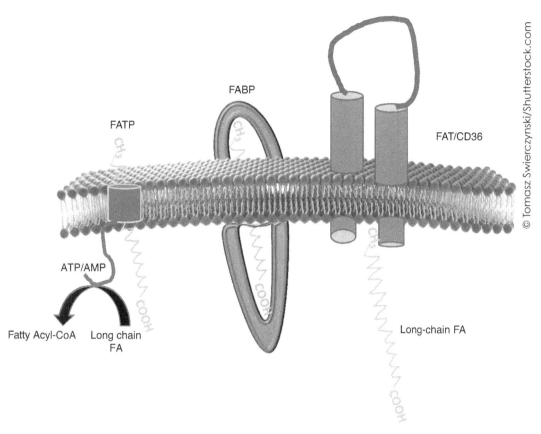

Figure 6.11: **Receptor-mediated Uptake of Fatty Acids.** Both FAT/CD36 and FABP have external membrane domains that can bind long chain fatty acids and transport them into the cell. FATP appears to sit inside the membrane, trapping long chain fatty acids (LCFAs) as they interact with the membrane. FATP has endogenous fatty acyl CoA synthetase activity, converting LCFAs to fatty acyl CoA molecules. FAT/CD36 and FABP appear to have both membrane bound and cytosolic forms. Like GLUT4, FAT/CD36 is translocated to the plasma membrane upon insulin-stimulation.

it is present in the liver at high levels[19]. FABP1 can bind to two separate molecules of long-chain fatty acids, and with both a membrane-bound, and cellular form, transport them into the cell. There, it appears to mediate trafficking of fatty acids as well as other molecules, even interacting with peroxisome proliferator activating receptors (PPARs), which mediate gene expression[19]. FABP proteins use 10 beta sheets to form what is known as a beta-barrel, which serves as a cavity for fatty acids to bind[19] (Figure 6.11). The last fatty acid transport protein is actually called "fatty acid transport protein" (FATP), which makes it easy to remember. This transport protein family has six members belonging to the solute carrier protein family #27A1–6 (SLC27)[20]. All of the FATP family members appear to be transmembrane proteins (Figure 6.11), which bind fatty acids as they interact with the cell membrane, converting them to fatty acyl CoA molecules on the other side through its inherent fatty acyl-CoA synthetase activity[21].

These three fatty acid receptors/transporters appear to be the most prominent transporters for the long- and some medium-chain fatty acids. Different tissue types express different isoforms of the protein families, and as we discussed for FAT/CD36 and FABP, there are both membrane and cytoplasmic forms of the proteins. On the other hand, the short-chain fatty acids are pretty much on their own and can diffuse into cells without additional transport proteins. At this point, once in the cells, fatty acids can be metabolized, stored, or used in signal transduction and gene expression pathways.

Protein Absorption, Transport and Recycling

Protein Digestion and Absorption

Other than chewing to get proteins out of the foods, there is no enzymatic digestion of protein in the mouth. So, let's move right to the stomach, where the real work begins, and some of the enzymes (Table 6.3) are located. Gastric acid, which is composed of hydrochloric acid (HCl) and the other enzymes and water in the stomach, has a pH of 1–2—extremely acidic, in other words, this acidic environment is the first method by which protein breakdown occurs. Remember though that proteins are usually folded into 3D structures, or even part of multi-protein structures—all of this has to be broken down before pepsin can work its wonders, and here is where that acidic environment can help. The acidic environment of the stomach breaks down 3D structure of proteins (also called "denaturation"). In addition, the enzyme pepsinogen, which is secreted by the chief cells of the stomach, actually utilizes this acidic environment to become activated. When pepsinogen is secreted into the gastric juices, the acid environment along with auto-enzymatic activity (i.e. it works on itself) result in activation of pepsinogen to the endopeptidase, pepsin. Pepsin is extremely important for protein breakdown as it is a nonspecific endopeptidase which can cleave proteins at multiple accessible locations (i.e. where it can gain access) within the middle of protein chains. The mixing that occurs (think stomach churning) aids in this enzymatic activity and allows for pepsin to get into the nooks and crannies of the protein and digest it. In particular, pepsin cleaves (hydrolyzes) peptide bones at the carboxy-side of aromatic amino acids (phenylalanine, tryptophan, and tyrosine)[22]. As the stomach empties, not all proteins are fully digested, but rather are a mix of single amino acids, short amino acid chains, and larger polypeptides.

The rest of protein digestion can be very complex because each protein is different, in 3D structure, in amino acid composition, and in overall charge (among other things). Within the small intestine, partial hydrolysis of proteins can break down proteins into small polypeptides. Unlike carbohydrates which have to be broken down to monosaccharides—their simplest form, some small polypeptides of just a few amino acids can be directly absorbed by the enterocyte. However, complete digestion of the proteins results in digestion of the protein to individual amino acids. Using specific enzymes and transporters, these amino acids can be individually taken up by the enterocyte. In the pancreas, proteolytic enzymes (those enzymes that can cleave proteins) are stored as zymogens, which are inactive forms of the enzymes. Storage as zymogens prevents inappropriate digestion of proteins (i.e. the wrong proteins, or at the wrong time). Once activated, they become proteases (also called proteinases and peptidases), and these proteases are the "business" enzymes for protein digestion, as they are able to cleave protein/amino acid bonds and release amino acids as well as short peptide chains from whole proteins.

As mentioned earlier, when the chyme slurry from the stomach enters the small intestine, two hormones are immediately released as well—cholecystokinin (CCK) and secretin. These hormones trigger the release of pancreatic juices and bicarbonate, respectively from the acinar cells of the pancreas. These pancreatic juices contain the proteolytic zymogens—trypsinogen, chymotrypsinogen, procarboxypeptidases, and proelastase, which are now released into the small intestine. However, these zymogens are not ready yet to digest protein because they need to be activated. How does this happen? Well, that hormonal stimulation also induces the activation of enteropeptidase, which is a brush border enzyme, located on the enterocytes. Enteropeptidase can cleave trypsinogen, forming trypsin. Trypsin can then activate the other zymogens to form chymotrypsin, carboxypeptidases, and elastase, and together all of these proteases can work to digest proteins. Putting it all together, Table 6.3 shows how each of the proteases recognized motifs and work to break down proteins.

Table 6.3: **Digestive proteolytic enzymes.**

Proteolytic enzyme	Pro-form	Secreted From	Activation	Target
Pepsin	Pepsinogen	Stomach mucosal chief cells	Auto/acidic pH	Cleaves between amino acids, to the C-terminus of Phe, Tyr, Trp
Trypsin	Trypsinogen	Pancreatic acinar cells	Enteropeptidase	Cleaves between Lys, Arg, to the C-terminus of each
Chymotrypsin	Chymotrypsinogen	Pancreatic acinar cells	Trypsin	Cleaves to Phe, Tyr, Trp, to the C-terminus of each
Carboxypeptidase A & B	Procarboxypeptidase A & B	Pancreatic acinar cells	Trypsin	C-terminal end amino acids (exopeptidase)
Aminopeptidases	none	Intestinal brush border cells	Requires ions such as zinc, calcium or chloride—different for each type	N- and C-terminal amino acids. Many different types of these enzymes target different amino acids

As you probably already imagined, peptidases are also found on the brush border of the small intestine. As the small intestine is composed of several functional areas—the duodenum, the jejunum, and the ileum, the peptidases are actually produced throughout each of the functional areas. Different types of aminopeptidases attack different types of peptides—aminopeptidases cleave from the end of a protein chain, cleaving off single amino acids; dipeptidases cleave from the end (N-terminus) of a dipeptide molecule, or one with two amino acids; tripeptidases cleave tripeptides, leaving one dipeptide, and one free amino acid—and many of these are specific to amino acid sequences.

Once all of the amino acids are liberated by the combination of proteases and peptidases, the amino acids are individually absorbed from the lumen of the small intestine, usually using amino acid-specific transferase receptors, some of which have overlapping specificity (Figure 6.12). These receptors are usually sodium dependent on the lumen side, although there are some that are sodium independent and many of these require energy in the form of ATP through secondary active transport (remember how SGLT1 worked? ATP is required to maintain the Na^+/K^+ balance in the cell). Interestingly, the majority of amino acid absorption takes place in the proximal small intestine (duodenum), although amino acid transferases are found throughout the brush border surfaces of the jejunum, and distal ileum.

The other complexity about amino acid absorption occurs due to the differential charges of amino acids, meaning that some amino acids are easier to absorb than others. For example, asparagine and glutamine, both having positive charges, have the slowest rate of absorption, while amino acids with more hydrocarbons, such as isoleucine, or those that are neutral (like alanine) will have a faster uptake. Take a look back at the list of amino acids and predict which ones will show slower versus faster uptake. Keep in mind that our body has also managed to preferentially facilitate the uptake of essential amino acids, as compared to non-essential amino acids. Remember the acronym

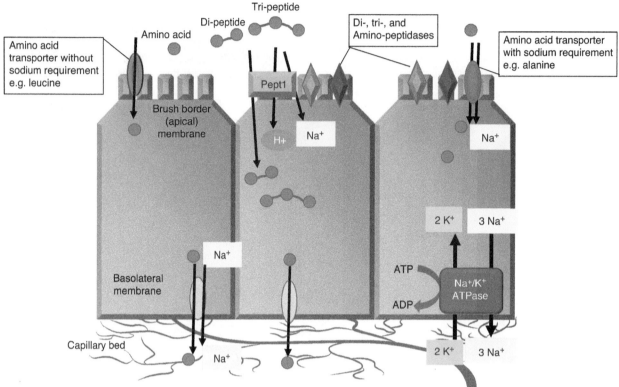

Figure 6.12: **Absorption of Digested Amino Acids and Peptides.** Aminopeptidases, dipeptidases, and tripeptidases on the brush border of the small intestine will digest short peptides forming tri- and di-peptides, as well as single amino acids. Amino acids and small peptides are absorbed by specific transporters, some of which require sodium or protons. This changes the sodium balance of the enterocyte, which must be fixed using the Na^+/K^+ ATPase to transport sodium back out to the capillaries (secondary active transport). Small peptides can be absorbed via the peptide transporter 1 (Pept1). Amino acid transporters on the basolateral membrane of the enterocyte transport amino acids out to the capillaries.

BEN—those that are big, essential, and/or neutral get absorbed over small, non-essential, and charged amino acids. In addition to individual amino acids, small peptides can be absorbed by a peptide transporter (PEPT1), which relies on a proton and sodium gradient system for transport (Figure 6.12). In fact, up to 67% of the protein that is absorbed is absorbed as small peptides, rather than individual amino acids. Once inside the enterocyte the peptides are broken down by cellular peptidases and then the amino acids are used for protein synthesis or transported out of the cell if not needed.

> **Viruses use amino acid transporters too**
>
> Some viruses, such as Coxackie virus, Karposi's sarcoma-virus associated herpes virus 8, and the virus causing yellow fever use amino acid transporters for entry into our intestine cells and then to our blood[23].

Amino Acid Transport and Recycling

As the amino acids are absorbed by intestinal cells or released by cellular peptidases following absorption of small peptides, they have two fates. One is that they can be transported across the basal-lateral membrane of the enterocyte into circulation (Figure 6.12), and the other is that they are used by the intestinal cell for its own protein synthesis. In fact, about 30–40% of the absorbed amino acids are never transported into circulation but are used by enterocytes directly. That's surprising in some ways, until you think

Table 6.4: **Amino acid and peptide transporters.** (A) Brush border transporters with alternate designations and type of transport (B) Basolateral transporters.

A.

Transporter	Designation (type)	Sodium	Amino Acids
L	Exchanger	No	Leu/neutral amino acids
B	Exchanger	Yes	Phe, Tyr, Trp, Ile, Leu, VAL
imino		Yes	Pro, Gly
Y^+/y	Facilitated	No/Yes	Basic and neutral amino acids
X^-_{AG}	Exchanger	Yes	Asp, Glu
B^+/b^+	Exchanger	Yes/No	Neutral amino acids
ASC/asc	Exchanger	Yes/No	Ala, Ser, Cys
N		Yes	Glu, Asp, His
ag	Exchanger	No	Asp, Glu

B.

Transporter	Sodium Requirement	Amino Acids
L	No	Leu/neutral amino acids
Y^+	No	Basic amino acids
$b^{a,+}$	No	Basic and neutral amino acids
t	No	Phe, Tyr, Trp
X^-_{AG}	Yes	Asp, Glu
A	Yes	Alanine, polar, neutral amino acids
ASC/asc	Yes/No	Ala, Ser, Cys
GLY	Yes	Gly

about the "lifespan" of an enterocyte. Enterocytes quickly turn over, and are sloughed off every 6 days, so enterocytes are making structural proteins for their own use all of the time and thus need this "free" source of amino acids. In addition, absorbed glutamine and glutamate are directly used by enterocytes for energy production, with their carbon chain feeding into the TCA cycle at alpha-ketoglutarate. Amino acids that are not needed by the enterocyte are shuttled out using specific amino acid transferases, most of which are sodium-independent transporters although some again use sodium as a co-transporter. All of these transferases can transfer amino acids in both directions (into and out of the cells), with the direction of transport depending on the needs of the cell. The specific amino acids transporters and the amino acids that are transported by them are listed in Table 6.4A, and Table 6.4B. Of note, different transporters have different affinities for amino acids, and unfortunately, somewhat odd designations (i.e. Y^+, B^+, X^-_{AG} and so on). One review paper divides these amino acid transporters into two main groupings—exchangers and facilitated diffusers, and Table 6.4A gives you these designations as well, if listed in the reference[23].

Amino acid transporters are generally exchangers, meaning that amino acids travel into and out of the cell through them (Figure 6.13). Yes, that is correct—recycling of amino acids occurs within cells, as proteins are degraded, and if not needed, amino acids transported back out to the amino acid pool in the plasma. Within a single cell, different proteins have different turnover rates, and within different cell and tissue types, overall protein turnout occurs at different rates. Let's look at this in more detail

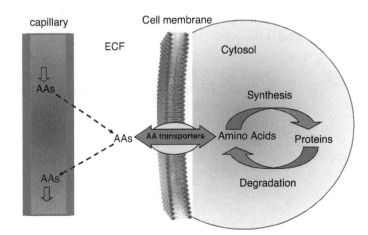

Figure 6.13: **Transport of Amino Acids between Cells and Circulation.** A conglomeration of different amino acid transporters (see Table 6.4) on the cell membrane are constantly picking up and releasing amino acids to balance cellular needs of protein synthesis with protein degradation.

with a few examples. Gastrointestinal tissue, which has a high cellular turnover rate, has a high protein synthesis rate, and high protein degradation rate. Conversely, the brain and even muscle, which have lower cellular turnover rates, have low protein synthesis rates and lower protein degradation rates[24]. In each, changes in demand can change protein synthesis and degradation rate, such that nothing is fixed, but rather fluid to what is going on in other tissues. It makes sense then that the liver, while having a generally high demand, can recycle some amino acids out into the plasma pool for transport to other tissues, such as small intestine, that might have additional needs. The amino acid pool of the body is always in a dynamic state with influx and efflux of amino acids to and from cells of the body.

Summary

As macro- (and micro-) nutrients move through the digestive system, the nutrients are absorbed and transported to the tissues that need them. When the resulting mixture moves into the large intestine, there is little left of value except some vitamins (like biotin and vitamin K, which are made by bacteria in the large intestine), short-chained fatty acids, and water. The large intestine absorbs these as needed, with the remaining feces excreted out of the body as waste. In the next section, we will consider the fates of the newly absorbed carbohydrates, fats, and proteins within the cell (the fed state).

Points to Ponder

➤ Choose a meal containing proteins, fats, and carbohydrates and consider the proportion of each macronutrients (and specific types of these) and trace the fates of each macronutrient type through the body to absorption.

➤ Take a look at online mendelian inheritance in man (OMIM https://omim.org/) and type "digestion" into the search box. What did you find? How do some of these conditions directly or indirectly impact macronutrient digestion? You can also type in specific enzymes and proteins to determine if they are affected by any genetic disease.

➤ How would surgical removal of any part of the digestive system impact macronutrient digestion and absorption? Consider the tongue, salivary glands, teeth, esophagus, stomach, pancreas, liver, gall bladder, and small intestine in your answer.

References

1. Perry GH, Dominy NJ, Claw KG, et al. Diet and the evolution of human amylase gene copy number variation. *Nat Genet.* 2007;39(10):1256–1260.

2. Peyrot des Gachons C, Breslin PA. Salivary Amylase: Digestion and Metabolic Syndrome. *Curr Diab Rep.* 2016;16(10):102.

3. Whitcomb DC, Lowe ME. Human pancreatic digestive enzymes. *Dig Dis Sci.* 2007;52(1):1–17.

4. Lu M, Li C. Nutrient sensing in pancreatic islets: lessons from congenital hyperinsulinism and monogenic diabetes. *Ann N Y Acad Sci.* 2018;1411(1):65–82.

5. Yan N. A Glimpse of Membrane Transport through Structures-Advances in the Structural Biology of the GLUT Glucose Transporters. *J Mol Biol.* 2017;429(17):2710–2725.

6. Thorens B. Central control of glucose homeostasis: the brain–endocrine pancreas axis. *Diabetes Metab.* 2010;36 Suppl 3:S45–49.

7. Thorens B, Mueckler M. Glucose transporters in the 21st Century. *Am J Physiol Endocrinol Metab.* 2010;298(2):E141–145.

8. Hand AR, Pathmanathan D, Field RB. Morphological features of the minor salivary glands. *Arch Oral Biol.* 1999;44 Suppl 1:S3–10.

9. Matczuk J, Zendzian-Piotrowska M, Maciejczyk M, Kurek K. Salivary lipids: A review. *Adv Clin Exp Med.* 2017;26(6):1021–1029.

10. Xiao X, Ross LE, Miller RA, Lowe ME. Kinetic properties of mouse pancreatic lipase-related protein-2 suggest the mouse may not model human fat digestion. *J Lipid Res.* 2011;52(5):982–990.

11. Wolska A, Dunbar RL, Freeman LA, et al. Apolipoprotein C-II: New findings related to genetics, biochemistry, and role in triglyceride metabolism. *Atherosclerosis.* 2017;267:49–60.

12. Cohn JS, McNamara JR, Schaefer EJ. Lipoprotein cholesterol concentrations in the plasma of human subjects as measured in the fed and fasted states. *Clin Chem.* 1988;34(12):2456–2459.

13. Fisher EA. The degradation of apolipoprotein B100: multiple opportunities to regulate VLDL triglyceride production by different proteolytic pathways. *Biochim Biophys Acta.* 2012;1821(5):778–781.

14. Hadjiphilippou S, Ray KK. Lipids and Lipoproteins in Risk Prediction. *Cardiol Clin.* 2018;36(2):213–220.

15. Zannis VI, Fotakis P, Koukos G, et al. HDL biogenesis, remodeling, and catabolism. *Handb Exp Pharmacol.* 2015;224:53–111.

16. Zhao L, Varghese Z, Moorhead JF, Chen Y, Ruan XZ. CD36 and lipid metabolism in the evolution of atherosclerosis. *Br Med Bull.* 2018.

17. Jain SS, Chabowski A, Snook LA, et al. Additive effects of insulin and muscle contraction on fatty acid transport and fatty acid transporters, FAT/CD36, FABPpm, FATP1, 4 and 6. *FEBS Lett.* 2009;583(13):2294–2300.

18. Pepino MY, Kuda O, Samovski D, Abumrad NA. Structure-function of CD36 and importance of fatty acid signal transduction in fat metabolism. *Annu Rev Nutr.* 2014;34:281–303.

19. Wang G, Bonkovsky HL, de Lemos A, Burczynski FJ. Recent insights into the biological functions of liver fatty acid binding protein 1. *J Lipid Res.* 2015;56(12):2238–2247.

20. Kazantzis M, Stahl A. Fatty acid transport proteins, implications in physiology and disease. *Biochim Biophys Acta.* 2012;1821(5):852–857.

21. Anderson CM, Stahl A. SLC27 fatty acid transport proteins. *Mol Aspects Med.* 2013;34(2–3):516–528.

22. Roberts NB. Review article: human pepsins - their multiplicity, function and role in reflux disease. *Aliment Pharmacol Ther.* 2006;24 Suppl 2:2–9.

23. Fotiadis D, Kanai Y, Palacin M. The SLC3 and SLC7 families of amino acid transporters. *Mol Aspects Med.* 2013;34(2–3):139–158.

24. Millward DJ, Garlick PJ. The pattern of protein turnover in the whole animal and the effect of dietary variations. *Proc Nutr Soc.* 1972;31(3):257–263.

CHAPTER 7

Carbohydrate Fates in the Fed State

Imagine at this point that we are in the fed condition, with the food we have eaten having been digested, absorbed, and transported. The nutrients are in the bloodstream. Now what? In this chapter we will talk about the possible fates for carbohydrates, and then in subsequent chapters we'll address possible fates for fats and proteins.

With glucose, there are multiple things that can happen, depending on the body's needs (Figure 7.1). Some of the glucose can be stored as glycogen or can be shuttled into glycolysis for ATP generation. Some of the glucose could go into the hexose monophosphate shunt (also called the Pentose Phosphate Pathway, or PPP), and some can go into the hexosamine biosynthetic pathway. Some glucose can also enter glycolysis but then be diverted to make glycerol or enter the TCA cycle but then diverted to make fatty acids. The type of tissue, as well as what is going on in the body as a whole, determines the ultimate fate of circulating glucose. For example, as shown in Figure 7.1, there are tissues that are obligatory users of glucose, meaning they must rely on glucose as a substrate of ATP production (through glycolysis) because they do not possess mitochondria (e.g. red blood cells). Other tissues like liver or

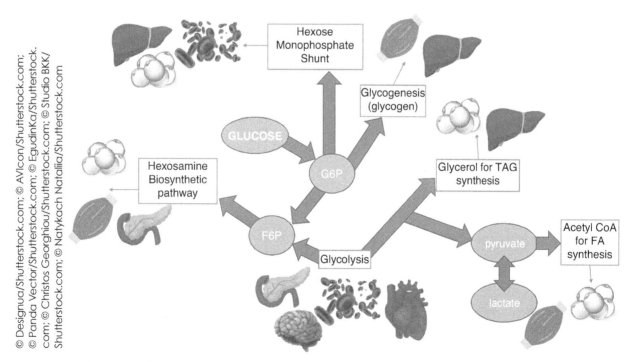

Figure 7.1: **Postprandial Fates of Glucose.** Glucose use or storage depends on several biochemical pathways, which are differentially active in the tissues receiving the glucose.

muscle might use the glucose directly or use glycogenesis to create glycogen from glucose so that it can be stored for later use. For liver, glycogenesis predominates. Adipose tissue might predominantly use glucose to produce acetyl CoA for *de novo* fatty acid synthesis, or produce glycerol for TAG synthesis, as well as use some for direct ATP production through glycolysis. The heart predominantly uses glucose in glycolysis to make ATP, which is why in Figure 7.1, that is the only place you see the heart.

Postprandial Fates of Glucose

One to three hours after your average meal of 500–1000 calories, energy storage is the predominate fate of the food taken in. You are in positive energy balance, but it is temporary, until you store or use the glucose and other macronutrients that have been taken in. But what happens in a person who is chronically in positive energy balance? And how does this person's metabolic usage of glucose compare to a person who is in negative energy balance, such as someone who is exercising, or dieting?

In a person who is chronically in a positive energy balance, their glycogen stores are likely full, and so glucose is likely not going to be diverted to glycogenesis, but rather to *de novo* fatty acid synthesis (Figure 7.2). In a person who is fed, but not in chronic positive energy balance, some glucose will be diverted to glycogen synthesis, but most of it will be used by regular cellular processes to generate ATP. In a person who has used their glycogen stores, such as someone who has just run a marathon, a lot of glucose will be diverted to make new glycogen and replenish the stored energy after using glucose for any additional needs.

The choice of fates is regulated by cellular signaling within the target tissues of the body. This will include both transcriptional (making new mRNA and proteins) and post-translational control (protein modification). Generally, the transcriptional mechanisms are in place to promote longer-term energy sensing and utilization. Both directly and indirectly, levels of circulating glucose or insulin released in response to glucose levels, will activate or repress transcription by using different transcription factors and gene targets. On the other hand, the

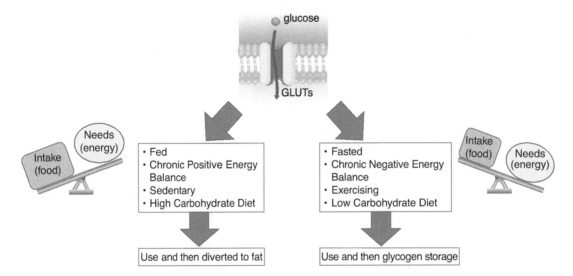

Figure 7.2: **Energy Balance and Glucose Fate.** Glucose uptake occurs via the glucose receptors (dependent on tissue type—see text), and its use is dependent on the specific needs of that tissue in relation to available food and energy. On the left, food intake is greater than energy needs, pulling down the teeter-totter. On the right, energy needs are greater than food intake, pulling down the teeter-totter.

post-translational mechanisms, which can be implemented and sensed within nanoseconds, are used for quick changes. These post-translational changes can be allosteric (shape-changing) or covalent (directly attached to proteins). Let's take a look at both of these more specifically.

Transcriptional and Post-translational Regulation of Carbohydrate Metabolism

Carbohydrate Sensing Transcription Factors

There are three main transcription factors that need to be considered when thinking about glucose metabolism: carbohydrate response element binding protein (ChREBP), sterol regulatory element binding protein (SREBP), and liver X receptor (LXR). Transcription factors generally bind to regions in the promoters of genes, usually at very specific DNA sequences (response elements), and in doing so, recruit other factors that result in the increase or decrease of transcription for that gene. This increase or decrease in transcription ultimately increases or decreases the amount of protein made from the mRNA of that gene. So right here, you can see that transcriptional regulation of carbohydrate metabolism requires a transcription factor binding to a spot in the DNA, changes in the transcription rate of DNA into mRNA, the amount of mRNA that is spliced and transported out to the cytoplasm for translation by ribosomes, and then the amount of protein folded into its active structure. Whew—that's a lot, right? So that is why transcriptional regulation of carbohydrate metabolism is more of a long-term regulatory process, rather than short term.

What genes do you think are targets of these transcription factors—ChREBP, SREBP, and LXR? Would you think these are genes that respond to the level of glucose in the bloodstream? No, probably not. We need quicker responses for that. Any increases and decreases in transcription rates are for our long-term responses, which include genes that regulate downstream metabolic pathways for carbohydrates—glycolysis, lipogenesis (the process of making lipid, either new fatty acids or TAGs) and glycogenolysis. Let's look at some of these in more detail.

The ChREBP transcription factor family are members of the basic helix-loop-helix/leucine zipper transcription factor family. These motifs allow ChREBPs to form heterodimers with other transcription factors to regulate activity. As a transcription factor, ChREBP binds to regions of the DNA called E-box motifs, CACGTG, to regulate gene expression in a glucose-dependent manner[1]. In fact, most promoters usually have two of these so-called carbohydrate-response motifs, separated by 5 random nucleotides[2]. With a name like "carbohydrate regulatory...", this transcription factor must be regulating carbohydrate metabolic genes, including some that you already know and should remember from previous chapters (or if you don't you will hear about them again). Only ChREBPα is induced by high glucose levels (Figure 7.3) and then

Genetics and ChREBP

ChREBP is deleted, along with about 26 other genes in a genetic syndrome called "Williams Syndrome". The condition is characterized by heart defects, and failure to thrive and gain weight in infancy. The patients also have myotonia, or low muscle tone. Some of these conditions could be caused by failure to properly metabolize carbohydrates but more research is needed to match the genotype with the phenotype of these individuals.

regulates a set of target genes. These gene targets include carbohydrate metabolism genes such as glycerol-3-phosphate dehydrogenase 1 (GPD1), glucose transporters GLUT2 and GLUT4,

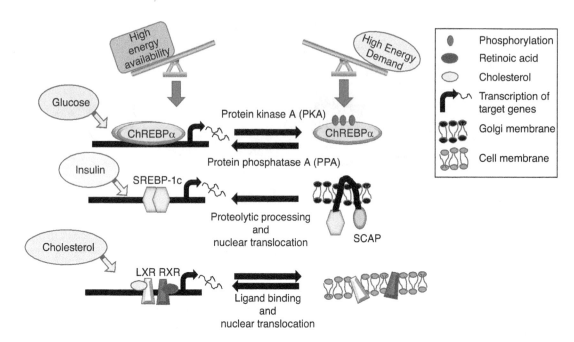

Figure 7.3: **Transcription Control of Carbohydrate Fates.** Allosteric (ligand binding), structural (proteolytic processing) and covalent (phosphorylation) regulation of transcription factors occurs in response to high or low energy demands.

glucose-6-phosphatase (catalytic subunit) (G6Pase), glucokinase/hexokinase (GK/HK), glucose-6 phosphate dehydrogenase (G6PDH), glucose-6-phosphate isomerase (GPI), fructokinase (FK), and pyruvate kinase (PK) which are all upregulated by ChREBPα[3]. ChREBPα even induces expression of its own gene, making more ChREBPα transcription factors[2]! The one gene associated with lipid oxidation that was examined in this study, Carnitine palmitoyltransferase 1 (CAT1—also known as carnitine palmitoyl transferase—CPT1), is significantly downregulated by ChREBPα[2], as are glucokinase (GK) and insulin (INS1, INS2)[3]. Modulation of ChREBPα activity is likely to change whether glycolytic or lipolytic pathways are induced, and as we will see momentarily, ChREBPα is the target of post-translational modifications which can alter its activity. Of note, ChREBPα, and ChREBPβ come from the same gene but use alternate promoters to create the two isoforms. ChREBPβ however, lacks a glucose-sensing domain and is constitutively active—not glucose regulated[3].

Sterol-regulatory element binding protein (SREBP), of which the most abundant form is SREBP-1c, is considered to be the most important transcription factor regulating carbohydrate metabolism in response to insulin[1]. There are two other isoforms, SREBP-1a, and SREBP-2 which we will not talk about. All family members have a very interesting regulatory pathway, involving sequestration within in the Golgi apparatus, proteolytic processing and nuclear translocation. However, only activation of the SREBP-1c isoform is induced by insulin in the liver[4]. All of this is done following a series of signaling events that occur after insulin binds. SREBP-1c is initially synthesized in a precursor form that stays in the endoplasmic reticulum, and is associated with both SREBP-1c cleavage activating protein (SCAP) and another protein called Insig[1]. The initial steps in SREBP-1c regulation involve sensing cellular cholesterol levels by the SREBP-SCAP-Insig complex. Small changes of just 5% can cause a conformational (allosteric) change in the protein complex such that the Insig protein is released, and SREBP-SCAP proteins migrate to the Golgi. Following insulin stimulation (which we will see later activates AKT kinase, and phosphatidylinositol-3-kinase- PI3K), SREBP-1c is proteolytically cleaved from SCAP, and it then migrates to the nucleus to transcribe target genes. SREBP-1c binds to the sterol regulatory element (SRE, TCACNCCAC, where "N" represents any nucleotide) which is found in the promoter regions of target genes involved in cholesterol metabolism, energy generation, and ketogenesis, including 3-Hydroxy-3-Methylglutaryl-CoA Reductase (*HMGCR,* for ketogenesis*)*, farnesyl pyrophosphate synthase (*FDPS,* which is needed for synthesis of CoQ in the electron transport chain*)*, and squalene synthase (*FDFT1,* for cholesterol biosynthesis*)*[5].

The last transcription factor in this group, although certainly not the least, is the liver X receptor (LXR). The name of this transcription factor comes from the fact that initially, the protein was thought to be a receptor for an unknown ligand. It was subsequently found that LXR is a member of the nuclear receptor family of transcription factors and binds to oxidized cholesterol derivatives. Normally LXR sits in the cell membrane (Figure 7.3), but upon binding to its ligand, LXR forms heterodimers with the retinoid X receptor, RXR, and translocates to the nucleus. There it activates gene expression of cholesterol and lipid metabolism genes, including ApoE, fatty acid synthetase (*FAS*), cholesterol 7α-hydroxylase (*CYPTa1*), and lipoprotein lipase (*LPL*), to name a few[6]. Interestingly, two of LXR's transcriptional targets are the transcription factors that we just discussed SREBP-1c, and ChREBP. Thus, high levels of oxidized cholesterol will lead to increased expression of genes involved in carbohydrate and cholesterol metabolism. This is important because unlike fatty acids, cholesterol cannot be degraded to acetyl CoA. Thus, LXR activation by cholesterol derivatives induces genes required for the entire process of reverse cholesterol transport leading to excretion.

Transcriptional Crosstalk

Just when you thought it was simply three transcription factors to worry about, more come along to complicate things. There are four other transcription factors that need to be mentioned, mainly for the cross-talk that occurs between them and SREBP1, ChREBPα, and LXR.

Peroxisome proliferator-activated receptors (PPARs) serve as molecular sensors of fat, protein, and carbohydrate energy sensing and metabolism. The three forms, PPARα (NR1C1, encoded by *PPARA*), PPARβ/δ (NR1C2, encoded by *PPARD*), and PPARγ (NR1C3, encoded by *PPARG*) are all members of the nuclear receptor transcription factor family (which actually includes at least 50 members)[7]. PPARs bind to polyunsaturated fatty acids, branched chain fatty acids, oxidized-fatty acids, phospholipids, in addition to other

> **A little fat does the body good**
>
> PPARγ whole body knockout mice lack the ability to make adipose tissue and a placenta. This results in death. Of interest, mice with just one PPARγ gene are protected from diet-induced obesity[8].

ligands and agonists. PPARs are considered "ligand activated" because binding to their ligand causes activation of the transcription factor, resulting in upregulation of the transcription of target genes such as fatty acid binding protein (FABP), acyl-CoA oxidase, fatty acid transport protein (FATP), GLUT4, carnitine palmitoyltransferase I (CPT1), and peroxisome proliferator-activated receptor gamma coactivator 1-alpha (PGC-1α)[7], another transcription factor that will be discussed below. PPARs do not act alone at the target gene promoter but require co-binding with retinoic acid nuclear hormone transcription factor, RXR (Figure 7.4). ChREBPs, whose activity is induced by glucose, is pro-adipogenic as well, leading to increased activation of PPARs in adipocytes by increasing interaction of PPARs with their ligands, fatty acids[9]. How does this occur? It appears to do so through ChREBP (both isoforms) stimulation of fatty acid synthetase (FAS) gene, which leads to synthesis of fatty acids, which acts as ligands for PPARα[9]. However, in pancreatic beta cells, and in the liver, negative regulation of PPARα occurs by ChREBP α (Figure 7.4). This becomes quite complicated fairly quickly, right? So, what's the bottom line? What researchers have concluded is that when there is excess glucose around,

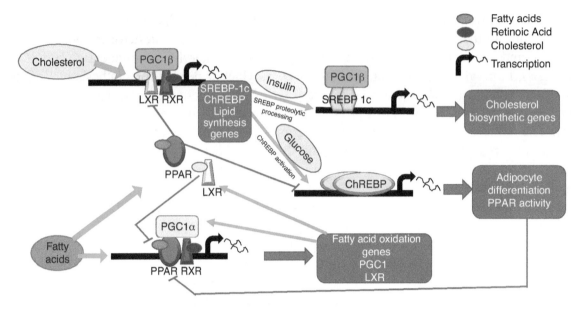

Figure 7.4: Transcriptional Cross-talk. As shown, cholesterol can stimulate LXR DNA binding, but LXR also leads to inhibition of PPAR DNA binding. PPAR transcription factors regulate (turn on) fatty acid oxidation genes, and importantly, induce expression of PCG1a, which initiates a positive regulatory loop of more PPAR activation. Activated PPAR/fatty acid complex can inhibit stimulation of LXR-regulated genes, such as SREBP-1c and ChREBP transcription factors. PPARs also turn on the LXR gene, leading to negative feedback on PPAR-regulated genes. See the chapter text for more information and references. PGC1b is a positive regulator of SREBP, ChREBP, and LXR transcriptional activity.

ChREBPα is stimulated as you would expect, and then it both stimulates fatty acid synthesis, but also, at least initially, fatty acid oxidation through PPARα-regulated genes. Eventually PPARα activity will turn off, as ChREBPα will also inhibit new transcription of the PPARα mRNA. This leads to fatty acid storage rather than oxidation. Don't forget there is also PPARγ, which is mainly found in adipocytes, as compared to PPARα mRNA, which is highest in liver, heart, and kidney. PPARδ is highest in skeletal muscle.

Enter your fourth transcription factor PPAR gamma-coactivator (PGC-1), which doesn't actually bind DNA, but acts as a co-activating protein (see Figure 7.4). The term again refers to a family of proteins, which include PGC1α, PGC1β, and at least two other factors which we will not discuss[10]. Each of these family members has a set of other transcription factors that they activate. For example, binding of PPARγ by PGC1α increases the transcriptional activity of PPARγ on its target gene promoters. In muscle cells, PGC1α expression is induced by PPARδ, and PGC1α is part of the muscle-cell's response to fasting, inducing fatty acid oxidation as one of its outcomes (see Figure 7.4)[11]. Similarly, PGC1β binds to both SREBP and ChREBP transcription factors, helping to mediate the response to carbohydrates in the liver by these transcription factors[11].

The cross-talk between these pathways are summarized in Figure 7.4, looking from the perspective of the main pathways, and generally, from the liver as the model. The main point is that carbohydrate and lipid sensing networks are coordinately regulated in the liver, adipose, muscle, and other metabolic-sensing tissues attempting to correctly respond to glucose, insulin, fatty acids, and cholesterol with the correct level of storage, biosynthesis, and energy generation pathways for each situation and in each tissue type.

While we just took a direct line to the nucleus and gene transcription, it is now time to step back and look at the signaling cascades which cause shorter-term changes, but which lead to these longer-term changes in gene and protein expression in the cells. Let's talk post-translational regulation!

Post-translational Regulation

Post-translational regulation involves rapid changes in response to signaling pathways, especially as compared to transcriptional regulation. These changes involve 1. allosteric regulation—or changes that occur via interaction of the enzyme with the substrate, intermediate product, or actual products of the enzyme, or 2. covalent regulation—involving changes directly on the enzyme, with the most common being phosphorylation of the enzyme.

Hexokinase—Transcriptional and Post-transcriptional (allosteric) Regulation

The enzyme hexokinase serves as the "gatekeeper" for glucose metabolism in nearly all metabolically active tissues and has both transcriptional and post-transcriptional regulation. This enzyme converts glucose into glucose-6-phosphate (G6P), using one molecule of ATP in the process. Once a cell has G6P, there are several options available for metabolism, and G6P is trapped in the cell at this point allowing for additional glucose uptake down its concentration gradient. Note that unphosphorylated glucose can diffuse out of the cell and go back into circulation. Thus, the phospho-

> **An enzyme by another name...**
>
> Hexokinase is the name this enzyme group goes by in most tissues—the exception is the pancreas and the liver, where the tissue-specific isoform goes by the name glucokinase. Keep this in mind, and you will recognize liver and pancreatic specific metabolic pathways.

rylation commits glucose to metabolism of some sort. As G6P accumulates, it can feed back and allosterically bind to hexokinase, inhibiting the enzymes activity (Figure 7.5a). This step is the first allosteric inhibition of glucose metabolism that occurs. There are four hexokinase isozymes, each encoded by different genes (*HK1, HK2, HK3, and GCK*) (Table 7.1)[12]. One of the most important differences between the different enzymes, in addition to their tissue specificity, is their K_m for glucose versus G6P[12]. But why have four different enzymes that essentially do the same thing—phosphorylate glucose—in the first place? It is thought that the four enzymes are required for fine tuning of glucose phosphorylation, with different concentrations of glucose, in different tissues, and in response to different metabolic states[12], and research into each of the enzymes has concluded that this is indeed the case (Table 7.1). Let's look at each hexokinase isoform individually, comparing and contrasting their activities towards both substrate and product, their tissue specificity, and response to different metabolic states.

The promoter regions of HK1-3 and glucokinase (GK) have been isolated and characterized, and it is clear that there is both tissue-specificity in expression, and in response to insulin levels[12]. HK1 is considered a "housekeeping" gene, and it is expressed by most tissues. As a housekeeping gene, it is not inducible by energy balance status or changes in insulin levels. Conversely, expression of GK (HK4/ GCK) is tissue-specific, with significant expression only in the liver, pancreas, and brain (neurons)[13] (Table 7.1). Interestingly, GK expression in liver and pancreas is under the control of two different regions of the promoter, resulting in different spliced mRNAs being produced in each tissue, leading to different GK isoforms[13]. The pancreatic beta cell specific isoform of GK regulates glucose-induced insulin secretion, while the liver-specific isoform of GK preferentially sends glucose-6-phosphate to the

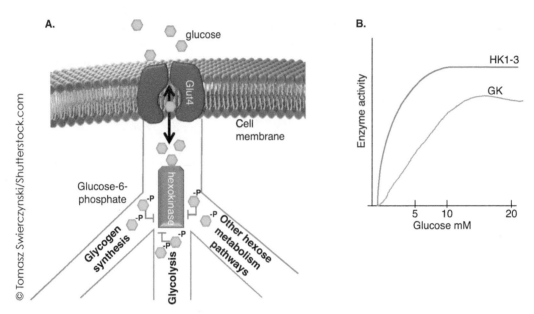

© Tomasz Swierczynski/Shutterstock.com

Figure 7.5: **Hexokinase—the Gatekeeper of Glucose Metabolism.** (**A**) Glucose can enter the muscle or liver cell via GLUT4 but this is not the defining step as glucose can still leave via GLUT4. Hexokinase (HK1-3, or GK) converts glucose into glucose-6-phosphate, permanently sealing its fate to a metabolic pathway within that cell type. High glucose-6-phosphate levels allosterically inhibit HK1-3 enzymatic activity (red bars). (**B**) The influx of glucose and concentration of glucose within a cell define the activity of the hexokinase family of enzymes. HK1-3 are enzymatically active only at low glucose levels, whereas GK requires higher levels to reach full activity.

Table 7.1: **Hexokinases 1–3 and Glucokinase.** Gene and protein name, tissue expression, enzymatic activity (K_m) in response to glucose, and regulation are shown.

ENZYME	GENE	TISSUE	mMol/l K_m(Glucose) K_m (G6)	Regulation
Hexokinase 1	HK1	Expressed in most tissues	0.03 0.02	Not regulated in most tissues G6P allosteric regulation
Hexokinase 2	HK2	Many tissues, predominant in muscle, adipose and heart	0.3 0.02	Insulin-inducible G6P allosteric regulation
Hexokinase 3	HK3	Bone marrow	0.003 0.1	Insulin-inducible G6P allosteric regulation
Glucokinase	GCK	Liver, Pancreas, Brain	5–10 >0.001	Insulin-inducible Not allosterically regulated by G6P levels

glycogen storage pathway[13]. Both of these forms, and the neuron form, are activated by very low concentrations of glucose (Table 7.1). GK in the brain is localized mainly to neurons in the energy-sensing areas of the hypothalamus, and like the pancreas, plays a role in glucose-sensing within these neurons[13].

The K_m of these enzymes is one of the key distinguishing features of HK1-3 versus GK (see Figure 7.5B). That is to say that the HK1-3 enzymes are active even when there are low glucose levels, whereas GK only becomes actives when glucose is above normal physiological levels (about 7 mM glucose).

Now, looking that the tissue-specific expression of these different hexokinase forms, it makes sense that high levels of glucose would cause insulin to be released by the pancreas, the brain to sense high energy availability, and for the liver to start making glycogen from the glucose to store the excess energy—right?

In addition, HK1-3 all can be allosterically-inhibited by higher levels of glucose-6-phosphate, which will shut down the enzyme in an allosteric fashion (Table 7.1); GK activity is not affected by glucose-6-phosphate levels. So how is GK regulated? It is regulated through interaction with another protein, glucokinase regulatory protein (GKRP)[14], especially in liver. In the liver, GKRP holds GK protein within the nucleus, until this interaction is disrupted by high glucose or high levels of fructose-1-phosphate (Figure 7.6). Then GK travels out to the cytoplasm to phosphorylate glucose[14]. This means that after a meal, GK is active and functioning to move glucose through glycogenesis and glycolysis. However, in a fasted state, GK will be held in the nucleus and unable to phosphorylate glucose. Taken together, this means that glycogenolysis and gluconeogenesis will be preferentially stimulated in the fasted state so that stores can be utilized with GK held in the nucleus, while storage will take place in the fed state with glycolysis and glycogenesis activity, when GK is active[14]. This is not true however in the pancreatic beta cells, or within the brain, where GK is not under the control of GKRP. Remember that the liver and the pancreas/brain express different isoforms—formed by differential-splicing of the mRNA for GK[13]. Let's take a look at the pancreatic and brain-specific regulation of GK.

GKRP is not expressed in pancreatic beta cells, and the pancreatic isoform of GK, while also maintaining the lower K_m for glucose, does not share the same function with liver GK. In the pancreatic beta cells, and in neurons, GK can modulate its own enzymatic activity, resulting in more or less G-6-P production in the cell[13]. All of this leads to more or less ATP production, which is the ultimate regulator in these tissues. The increasing ATP/ADP ratio causes depolarization of the membrane by closing ATP sensitive potassium channels, causing opening of voltage-sensitive calcium changes, leading to release of insulin (in beta cells) or neurotransmitters (in neurons)[15] (see chapter 6). But how do these cells "stop" GK from continuing glycolytic flux and ATP production releasing insulin or neurotransmitters during lower glucose times? Two proteins, midnolin, and parkin appear to control protein levels of GK in pancreas and brain. These proteins also appear to work in liver as a second pathway for regulating GK[16]. Both midnolin and parkin have ubiquitin ligase domains (ULD) that target proteins, such as (but not limited to) GK for degradation by cellular proteasomes (Figure 7.6). The ULD on midnolin and parkin direct ubiquitin ligase to add ubiquitin to the protein (in this case GK), sealing its fate and targeting it for proteasome degradation. Interestingly, mRNA transcription for both midnolin and parkin is turned on when glucose levels are low, leading to increased levels of midnolin and parkin in the cell[16]. While the exact mechanisms for midnolin and parkin gene expression in response to low glucose levels have not been described yet, it is likely due to post-translational regulation of transcription factors that ultimately control their expression.

To close, HK/GK represents a decision point for the cell, and as such there are multiple ways that it is regulated in response to both high and low glucose levels. These regulatory points are all post-translational in nature—at least for GK, as the protein is either quickly brought out to the cytoplasm (in the case of liver) or ubiquitinated and sent to the proteasome for degradation (in all three tissues), depending on energy needs and glucose availability. As for HK, high levels of G6P feedback on the pathway, decreasing its enzymatic activity.

> **Something to ponder**
>
> Mutation of either midnolin and parkin are associated with the age-associated condition, Parkinson's Disease. How or why does their activity in GK regulation have anything to do with neuron cell death?

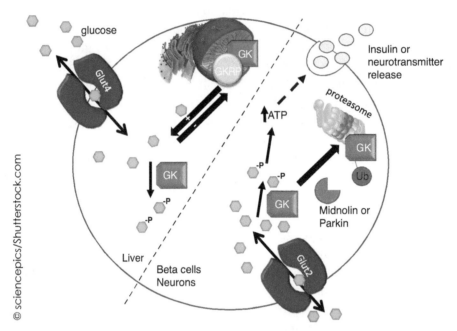

© sciencepics/Shutterstock.com

Figure 7.6: **Allosteric and Proteolytic Regulation of Glucokinase.** Unlike hexokinase which is regulated by glucose-6-phosphate levels, glucokinase (GK) is regulated by GK regulatory protein (GKRP) in the liver, and by proteolytic degradation, controlled through midnolin or parkin in pancreatic beta cells and neurons. Note that in beta cells and neurons, increasing glucose-6-phosphate leads to increased ATP and release of insulin (beta cells) or neurotransmitters (neurons).

Glycogenesis

We've talked a lot about glycolysis and the downstream pathway for energy generation, but now it is time to discuss another fate of glucose-6-phosphate and that is how we store some of that energy for later use. This is a particularly good time for us to do that, as the enzymes in glycogenesis are under post-translational control by kinases and phosphatases that regulate whether glycogen will be synthesized or broken down. At the center of this process lies the glycosome—a cellular organelle where glycogen is made and broken down. The raw materials such as glycogen itself, and glycogenin (the starting material), the enzymes glycogen synthase and glycogen phosphorylase, debranching and branching enzymes, and the kinases and phosphatases that regulate the process are all contained within the glycosome.

> **Did you know?**
> Unlike glycosomes in trypanosomes and some other protozoa, glycosomes in animals are not surrounded by lipid membranes. Because of this distinction, scientists are trying to develop drugs to target the glycosomes of trypanosomes, as these organisms cause the blood-borne diseases sleeping sickness and Chagus Diease.

As mentioned above, glycogenin is the molecule that starts it all. It is actually an enzymatic protein with the ability to add up to 7 glucose molecules to its end, and thus is a member of the glycosyltransferase enzyme family—enzymes that transfer glucose molecules. Once ~7 glucose molecules have been added to the end of glycogenin, glycogen synthase can take over and begin adding more glucose using α1-4 glycosidic bonds. Approximately every 13 glucose molecules, the branching enzyme then adds 7 additional glucose modules using a "branched"

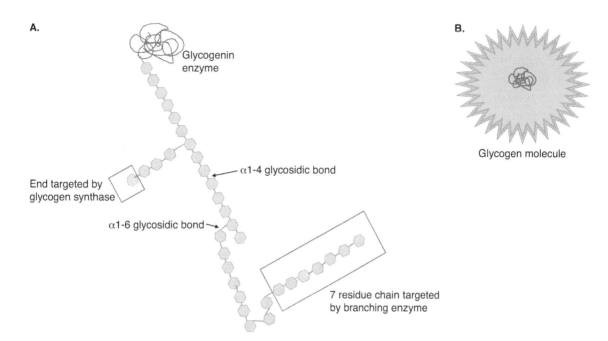

A.

Glycogenin
enzyme

α1-4 glycosidic bond

End targeted by
glycogen synthase

α1-6 glycosidic bond

7 residue chain targeted
by branching enzyme

B.

Glycogen molecule

Figure 7.7: **Glycogen.** Glycogen is composed of a molecule of glycogenin (**A**), linked to glucose molecules either in linear chains linked by α1-4 bonds, or branched through α1-6 bonds. Glycogenin starts the process by adding up to 7 glucose molecules directly to it's end. Glycogen synthase adds the α1-4 linear bonds, while the branching enzyme takes 7 residue chains of glucose, and adds it to a linear chain via an α1-6 bond. (**B**) The glycogen molecule, through both linear and branched glucose is highly compact, with a glycogenin enzyme at its center.

α1-6 glycosidic bond. These 7 glucoses come by cutting off of one of the growing chains and transferring it to the branch site (Figure 7.7). By doing this, the glycogen molecule is compact, with both straight and branched chains emanating from the original glycogenin enzyme. Let's step back for a moment, because the glucose that is used for glycogen synthesis is not glucose itself, or even G6P. Rather it is UDP-glucose, which is formed following conversion of G6P to G1P using phosphoglucomutase, and then transfer of a UDP moiety from uridine triphosphate (a nucleotide for RNA synthesis!) via UDP-glucose pyrophosphorylase. Glycogen synthase (GS) adds the UDP-glucose molecule to the growing glycogen chain, leaving behind the UDP. There are actually two forms of glycogen synthase—one for the liver and one for muscle and other tissues. These two forms are encoded by two different genes, and thus, as you might imagine, are under different transcriptional regulation. However, post-translational regulation is similar, and is what we need to discuss next.

As you might have guessed, glycogen synthase (GS) is active when glucose levels are high, and energy needs were low. Conversely, glycogenolysis, catalyzed by glycogen phosphorylase (GP) is high when glucose levels are low, but energy needs are high. This is true, but how is it regulated? Post-translational modification, and in the case of GS and GP—through covalent modification (addition or removal) of a molecule of phosphate to each protein—this is where the process gets sort of neat! Remember that depending on the conditions—high energy/low energy high demand/low demand, decisions must be made to determine if glucose is needed (glycogenolysis), used immediately (glycolysis), or stored (glycogenesis). These decisions need to be made quickly, and thus, both allosteric regulation and covalent regulation of enzymes are used.

Covalent Regulation of Glycolysis, Glycogenolysis, and Glycogenesis

As we mentioned above, glycogen synthase (GS) and glycogen phosphorylase (GP) are part of the glycosome. As such, at any given time, and depending on energy needs, there needs to be ways to turn one enzyme off and another enzyme on quickly. This is where covalent modifications, namely in the form of phosphorylation and dephosphorylation occur. It's complicated but let's take a look at Figure 7.8, which should help you to visualize what is going on in response to signals of insulin, glucose, and glucagon bombarding the cell (at different times!). Note that this figure and the description below, is most relevant to the liver, and then to the muscle.

The liver and skeletal muscle store glucose in the form of glycogen so that glucose can be released in times of need such as fasting, especially in the liver, and during exercise in skeletal muscle. When glucose is abundant, the pancreas will release insulin. Insulin binds to its receptor, the insulin receptor and catalyzes autophosphorylation of itself—activating the downstream molecule—insulin receptor substrate 1 (IRS1). This causes activation of one kinase (covalently adds phosphate), and one phosphatase (removes covalently attached phosphate). The activated kinase is phosphoinositol-3-kinase (PI3K), while the phosphatase is protein phosphatase 1 (PP1) (Figure 7.8)[17]. P13K targets the kinase AKT (also sometimes referred to as protein kinase B or PKB), which phosphorylates glycogen synthase kinase-3 (GSK-3), inhibiting it. This means that glycogen synthase is not being phosphorylated. PP1 is also removing any phosphates attached to GS, so in conjunction with the blocking of GSK and the activity of PP1, GS is active, leading to glucose storage. PP1 also removes the phosphates from GP, rendering it inactive, meaning that glycogenolysis will not occur. So here with just a few steps, we have the simultaneous turning on of glycogenesis and turning off of glycogenolysis.

Conversely, when one is fasted, and blood glucose levels need to be maintained, glucagon is released from the pancreas, and this initiates a different pathway which ultimately stimulates glycogenolysis (and gluconeogenesis, which will be discussed later) and inhibits glycogenesis. With

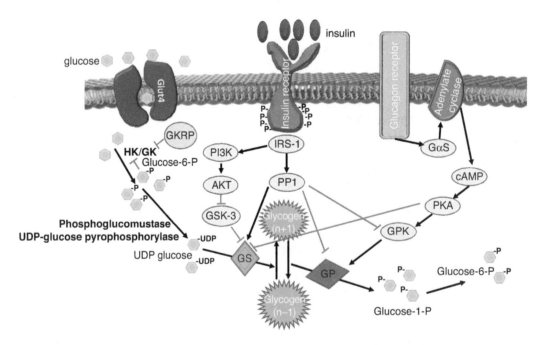

Figure 7.8: **Signals Mediating Regulation of Glycogenesis and Glycogenolysis.** The responses to insulin or glucagon differentially induce pathways to stimulate or inhibit glycogen synthase and glycogen phosphorylase, resulting in the breakdown or synthesis of glycogen, respectively. See text for abbreviations.

glucagon stimulation, phosphorylation of glycogen synthase (GS) on serine residues (amino acids) occurs via protein kinase A (PKA), and glycogen synthase kinase-3 (GSK-3)[17]. When GS is phosphorylated (covalent modification), it is inactive. However, the opposite is true for glycogen phosphorylase (GP). It is also the target of kinases and phosphatases as you can see in Figure 7.8. When GP is phosphorylated, it is active, and it is targeted by a kinase called glycogen

> ### Did you know?
> Calcium is the fifth most abundant element in the earth's crust, but the most abundant mineral in our body. This is due to both its role in the skeletal system, and in cellular signaling.

phosphorylase kinase (GPK), which itself is a target of PKA. Note also that PP1, which is removing phosphates from GP and rendering it inactive when energy is plentiful (insulin stimulation) is not at all activated by the glucagon pathway, which again make sense and keeps GP active. All of these covalent modifications, starting from insulin receptor, and continuing through GP and GS can occur in a matter of seconds to minutes—and are much faster than transcription of new proteins in response to extracellular signals. In addition, adding and removing phosphates can switch proteins on and off without having to "waste" materials by degrading them and then remaking new proteins. Again, cellular physiology amazes us with its conservation and recycling mechanisms.

Before leaving this topic, we need to talk about two more kinases that are involved in glucose metabolism in liver (and skeletal muscle)—AMP kinase (AMPK) and calmodulin kinase kinase (CaMKK). Let's start with CaMKK. As you have seen before, calcium signaling, either through the opening of intracellular stores from the endoplasmic reticulum, or influx through calcium channels, is one of the most important and utilized signaling pathways for cells. So, bearing this in mind, it should be of no surprise that we see calcium signaling in response to glucose uptake. One of the main targets of calcium is the calcium-binding protein calmodulin (CaM). CaM can bind up to 4 calcium molecules, which affects the conformation of CaM, rendering it activated. Activated CaM binds to many different

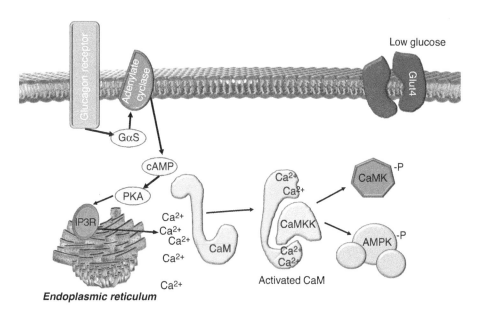

Figure 7.9: **Calcium Signaling and Gluconeogenesis.** Glucagon, through its receptor stimulates a signaling pathway that leads to calcium release from the endoplasmic reticulum. Calcium binds to and activates Calmodulin (CaM) which in turn activates Calmodulin kinase-kinase (CaMKK). Activated CaMKK can phosphorylate CaMK and AMPK.

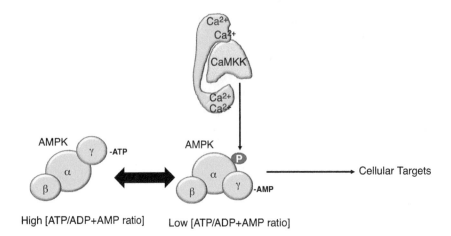

High [ATP/ADP+AMP ratio]   Low [ATP/ADP+AMP ratio]

Figure 7.10: **AMPK Regulation of Gluconeogenesis.** When ATP is plentiful, it is bound to AMPK γ subunit. However, as ATP supplies get lower, AMP and ADP compete for binding, allosterically changing the conformation of AMPK, such that the catalytic domain is exposed for phosphorylation (P) by CAMKII.

targets within the cell, including for the purpose of this discussion, CaMKK (Figure 7.9)[18]. CaMKK, as the name suggests, can phosphorylate CaM kinase (CaMK), but also AMPK. Both of these are important in downstream regulation of glucose homeostasis, but perhaps more so, AMPK. This signaling pathway is activated when there is higher energy demand and/or low glucose. Glucagon binding to its receptor causes activation of adenylate cyclase, and cAMP formation, followed by PKA activation and phosphorylation of the inositol triphosphate (IP_3) receptor (IP3R) on the endoplasmic reticulum, which stabilizes it in the open position. At the same time a second G-coupled receptor (possibly due to catecholamine binding), can activate phospholipase C (PLC) which produces IP_3 and a diglyceride (DAG) from the phospholipid—phosphatidylinositol 4,5-bisphosphate (PIP2). IP_3 then binds to the phosphorylated IP_3R, which causes a wave of calcium release from the endoplasmic reticulum, activating CaM by binding and causing a conformational (allosteric) change. CaM is now ready and able to bind to CaMKK, which leads to phosphorylation of both CaMK, and AMPK[18,19].

AMPK is a biological sensor of energy status in many tissues. Focusing on the liver and skeletal muscle, when the [ATP/ADP+AMP] ratio is low, meaning there is more ADP and AMP in the cell than ATP. AMPK is allosterically semi-activated by AMP binding to its γ-domain, opening up the catalytic domain for phosphorylation by CaMKK (Figure 7.10). This fully activated AMPK phosphorylates many different proteins, including those involved in lipid metabolism (e.g. ACC1), transcription (e.g. PGC1α), and glucose regulating pathways (e.g. Fructose-2,6-Biphosphatase)[20]. Recent work using mice with a targeted deletion of AMPK suggests that AMPK does not directly activate gluconeogenesis in the liver, but rather increases TCA cycle flux, and production of ATP[21]. This helps the liver to continue to make ATP needed for cellular processes, like gluconeogenesis. This bring us to another regulatory point in carbohydrate metabolism-fructose metabolism.

Fructose Metabolism—Another Regulatory Point

Let's revisit glycolysis again to review the points at which glucose or downstream substrates can enter glycolysis. As shown on Figure 7.11, glucose enters at the start of glycolysis, while glucose coming from glycogenolysis in the liver, is in the form of glucose-6-phosphate, and thus enters at the second step of glucose. Foods also contain fructose and galactose simple sugars, and as we have seen earlier, these can be absorbed by the intestine, and then by tissues. Fructose is absorbed and excreted by using

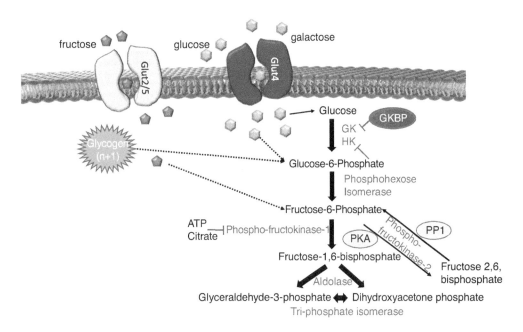

Figure 7.11: **Glycolysis, Revisited**. Glucokinase (hexokinase), phosphofructokinase-1, and phosphofructokinase II are all subject to covalent and/or allosteric regulation.

either GLUT5 or GLUT2, while both glucose and galactose use GLUT4 for absorption. Fructose can be phosphorylated by fructokinase in the liver, and then enters glycolysis either as fructose-6-phosphate, or later down, with a few more conversions as glyceraldehyde-3-phosphate. Note that by entering at these two downstream steps, fructose metabolism saves either one (when entering as fructose-6-phosphate) or two (when entering as glyceraldehyde-6-phosphate) ATP-requiring steps, as compared to starting with glucose. This makes use of fructose more energetically efficient-right? But what are the consequences of a high-fructose diet? Multiple reviews of the literature suggest that high-fructose diets contribute to metabolic syndrome, and fatty liver disease (for example, [22]), perhaps due to the increase energy that can be made relative to glucose, or perhaps due to other factors. Certainly, both ATP and citrate concentrations allosterically inhibit PFK-1 (Figure 7.11), as increases in these signal that energy needs are being met. By entering glycolysis below this regulatory step, fructose metabolism is not regulated by energy demand. In addition, as fructose does not use GLUT4 which is housed intracellularly until stimulated by insulin binding, there is no insulin regulation to fructose's uptake, as there is glucose. This leaves the control of fructose metabolism mainly to the liver. Let's look at this in more detail.

More than 35 years ago, the molecule fructose 2, 6, bisphosphate was discovered. You might be thinking—but that isn't an intermediate in glycolysis, and you are correct. It isn't an intermediate in any biochemical carbohydrate metabolic pathway that has been discovered yet, but it is used in the switch between glycolysis and gluconeogenesis[23]. This molecule is a very potent, positive allosteric regulator of 6-phosphofructo-1-kinase (PFK-1) and an inhibitor of fructose-1,6-bisphosphatase (FBPase-1). A single enzyme, called 6-phosphofructo-2-kinase or fructose 2,6-bisphosphatase (PFK-2 or FBPase-2, we'll refer to it as PFK-2) makes and degrades fructose 2,6 bisphosphate[23] (Figure 7.11). Phosphorylation of PFK-2 by PKA inhibits the enzyme, making less fructose 2,6 bisphosphate, while removal of the phosphate by PP1 causes increased production of fructose 2,6 bisphosphate[23]. As fructose 2,6 bisphosphate allosterically activates PFK-1, high levels will drive glycolysis and block gluconeogenesis in the liver. You can see that both PKA and PP1 act in these same metabolic pathways for pyruvate kinase also (see below), so that it all comes

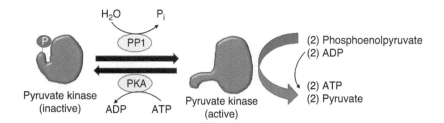

Figure 7.12: **Pyruvate Kinase Regulation**. Phosphorylation of pyruvate kinase (PK) on Serine #12 by PKA causes a conformational change that blocks the substrate binding domain. Removal of the phosphate group by PP1 leads to PK activation and continuation of glycolysis, yielding 2 pyruvate and 2 ATP molecules from one molecule of glucose.

together and makes sense. In addition to glycolysis/gluconeogenesis, we see that PKA and PP1 are also active in regulating glycogenesis and glycogenolysis (refer back to Figure 7.8).

There is one last regulatory point that needs to be addressed before we move on, and that is the regulation at pyruvate, through pyruvate kinase (PK). First, accumulation of fructose 1,6 bisphosphate will feed forward and allosterically activate PK. But the main regulation comes through the covalent attachment and removal of phosphate groups—catalyzed by PKA and PP1, respectively (Figure 7.12)[24]. Phosphorylated PK is inhibited because the phosphorylation of serine amino acid #12 causes a block of the substrate binding area for PK. Thus, when PKA is active (again refer to Figure 7.8) following glucagon stimulation or when energy needs are being met, PK activity is inhibited, providing a block at the last step of glycolysis, and preventing the production of 2 pyruvate and 2 additional molecules of ATP (Figure 7.12). It is important to note that this regulatory step only takes place in liver, and not in muscle. In muscle, levels of ATP, citrate, and free fatty acids directly allosterically inhibit PK activity, and like the liver, levels of fructose 1,6, bisphosphate allosterically activate PK.

Glyceroneogenesis

Before leaving glycolysis, we need to discuss the branch point at the fructose 1,6 bisphosphate step, namely, the enzymatic step catalyzed by aldolase (see Figure 7.11). Glycerol can be synthesized when there is incomplete or partial hydrolysis of fructose 1, 6 bisphosphate by aldolase to dihydroxyacetone phosphate (DHAP), rather than glyceraldehyde-3-phosphate (G3P). DHAP can then be converted into glycerol-3-phosphate by glycerol phosphate dehydrogenase. As glycerol-3-phosphate forms the

> **Are you allergic to fish or shellfish?**
>
> If so, it might be due to an IgE response to the fish/shellfish aldolase enzyme! See the review by Hilger and colleagues for more information[25].

backbone of triglycerides, this pathway can lead to higher triglyceride levels. Interestingly, aldolase is bound to the cytoskeleton of cells (and inactive) when ATP needs are being met. This is done through PI3K phosphorylation of aldolase, which causes it to interact with (bind) actin and become inactivated[26]. Note that in Figure 7.8, PI3K is upstream in the signaling pathway to activate glycogen synthase as well, diverting glucose-6-P to glycogen. Thus, the ultimate result of this will be a slowing down of glycolysis (if ATP demands are met), and when glycerol formation is favored, aldolase is no longer sequestered, and conversion of DHAP to glycerol-3-phosphate occurs.

De Novo Fatty Acid Synthesis

De novo fatty acid synthesis following carbohydrate ingestion can take place (and does!!) all of the time, but there are specific times when the process is ramped up. These include states of high calorie intake, high carbohydrate diets, conditions that increase insulin concentrations in the blood, and the general fed state (as opposed to a fasting state). On the other hand, *de novo* fatty acid synthesis would be low when there is a negative calorie balance—with more energy going out than coming in, high fat diets, and any time when you don't need to synthesize fatty acids, since there are ample amounts present in the diet that are being absorbed. Low insulin levels would also slow down *de novo* fatty acid synthesis.

Regulation of *de novo* fatty acid synthesis can be short term or long term. We've just talked about some conditions that can affect this, so let's look at the molecules that signal these changes. In the short term, accumulation of citrate in the TCA cycle will cause citrate to be shuttled out of the mitochondria and increase the production of malonyl CoA in the cytoplasm. Malonyl CoA increases *de novo* fatty acid synthesis due to a positive allosteric effect on acetyl CoA carboxylase (ACC1). ACC1 can be turned off by covalent modifications, such as phosphorylation by the kinases AMPK and PKA. Remember that both of these kinases are activated when energy demands are high or when the cells are stressed and need to make ATP—so this makes perfect sense because in these situations we would want to be using glucose and acetyl CoA to feed into the TCA cycle, rather than synthesizing fatty acids for storage. When ACC1 is phosphorylated, fatty acid synthesis will be shut down. Conversely, removal of the phosphate group by protein phosphatase 4 (related to PP1, which we have discussed previously), promotes fatty acid synthesis[27]. We also have longer-term regulation of fatty acid synthesis, and by this, we mean that gene expression of fatty acid synthetase, ACC1, ATP citrate lyase, malic enzyme (for producing NADPH) and all of the pentose phosphate enzymes, can be modulated transcriptionally to either increase or decrease fatty acid synthesis.

> **Food for thought...**
>
> If a high fat diet is being consumed, does the body synthesize fats—why or why not?

But let's go back to pyruvate for a minute. At this point, acetyl CoA is being formed, but it is in the mitochondria. We have to get acetyl CoA out of the mitochondria to even consider making fatty acids. This process of transport of acetyl CoA out of the mitochondria is called the citrate shuttle (Figure 7.13). Acetyl CoA enters the TCA cycle where it combines with oxaloacetate to make citrate via citrate synthase. Citrate is then shuttled out of the mitochondria in exchange for malate via the citrate transport protein (CTP). Citrate is cleaved back to oxaloacetate and acetyl CoA in the cytoplasm. Oxaloacetate is converted to malate by malate dehydrogenase (MDH). Back inside the mitochondria, the reverse reaction takes place and malate is converted back to oxaloacetate, allowing the TCA cycle to continue. Did you notice that? In order to transport acetyl CoA, we have to form citrate, through the action of citrate synthase, and then reconvert the citrate back to oxaloacetate and acetyl CoA. This second reaction is catalyzed by ATP-citrate lyase (ACL) and it requires ATP, as indicated by the enzyme. Now, malonyl CoA synthesis from acetyl CoA requires a bicarbonate molecule to donate the third carbon to make malonyl CoA. The enzyme that performs this function is called acetyl CoA carboxylase 1, or ACC1. As shown on Figure 7.13, ACC1 is one of the regulatory points in this process, and as discussed above, it is either inhibited or activated by the covalent attachment or removal, respectively, of a phosphate group.

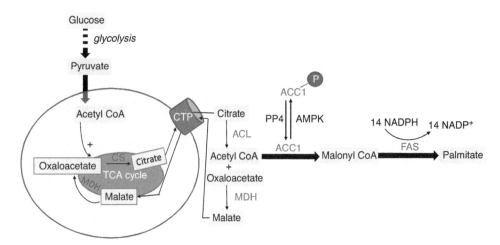

Figure 7.13: **ACC1 and the Citrate Shuttle.** High acetyl CoA levels can be shuttled out of the mitochondria using the citrate shuttle. Acetyl CoA needs one molecule of oxaloacetate to be converted to citrate in the TCA cycle, which can be shuttled out to the cytoplasm in exchange for malate using the citrate transport protein (CTP). The supply of oxaloacetate comes from a recycling of the citrate by acetyl CoA lyase (ACL) (+ 1 ATP), which forms acetyl CoA and oxaloacetate. The oxaloacetate can be converted to malate by malate dehydrogenase (MDH) and shuttled back into the mitochondria. ACC1 is a regulatory point for *de novo* fatty acid synthesis from acetyl CoA. When phosphorylated by PKA, ACC1 is inactive. When protein phosphatase 4 (PP4) removes the phosphate group, ACC1 becomes active and converts acetyl CoA to malonyl CoA, which can be used by fatty acid synthetase (FAS) to make palmitate. 14 NADPH molecules are consumed during fatty acid synthesis.

So, as you can see, carbons of glucose can be used to make fats—and this occurs especially when there are left-over glucoses. This process occurs mainly in "lipogenic" tissues, such as adipose, liver, and mammary glands, but really can occur in any tissue that has mitochondria. What this means is that when excess glucose is consumed, especially when there is low energy demand in that tissue, *de novo* fatty acid synthesis can occur. Rates are going to be highest in those tissues that are lipogenic, as mentioned above, but will occur in other tissues when there is chronic intake of excess glucose.

To review, we need to have excess acetyl CoA that is produced from glycolysis but isn't needed for the TCA cycle. Acetyl CoA then is shuttled into *de novo* fatty acid synthesis. Thus, acetyl CoA has two functions—to start the process of fatty acid synthesis, and to produce malonyl CoA, which is the carbon donor for fatty acids, via acetyl CoA carboxylase (ACC1). There are actually two forms of the ACC enzyme—both produce malonyl CoA, but the fate of the malonyl CoA produced from ACC1 versus ACC2 is different. ACC1 is the enzyme that is important for fatty acid synthesis and is found in the tissues that have a high capacity for making fatty acids, such as adipose tissue and liver. ACC2 on the other hand is important for the regulation of beta-oxidation of fatty acids in the mitochondria—a process that might occur more in skeletal muscle than adipose, and one that we will discuss later.

Genetic variation affects ability to eat fava beans

Some people cannot eat fava beans, due to a mutation which inactivates or reduces enzymatic activity of G6PD. This condition, called favism, can be deadly, and result in hemolysis of red blood cells when fava beans are consumed. Most newborns are tested for the condition, although the condition is more prevalent in individuals of Middle Eastern and northern African descent than other ethnic groups. Of note, mutations in G6PD can protect individuals from malaria, which may be why the mutation is prevalent in regions where malaria is present.

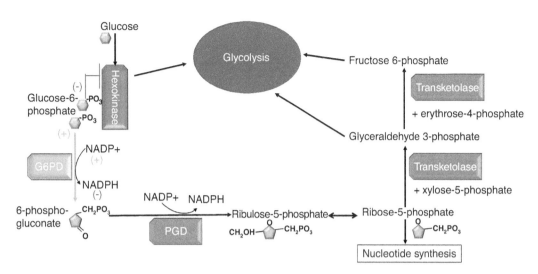

Figure 7.14: **The Hexose Monophosphate Shunt (Pentose Phosphate Pathway)**. Glucose-6-phosphate can be shuttled to the pentose phosphate pathway (PPP) during low energy needs, or when NADP$^+$ levels are high. The first two steps of the PPP are not reversible. High NADP$^+$ or G6P levels can drive the glucose-6-phosphate dehydrogenase enzyme, while high NADPH levels will allosterically inhibit the enzyme. 6-phospho-gluconate dehydrogenase (PGD) completes the second step, forming more NADPH, and ribulose-5-phosphate, which can be converted into ribose-5-phosphate, a direct precursor for nucleotide synthesis. Ribose-5-phosphate can also be further converted into glyceraldehyde 3-phosphate by the enzyme transketolase, which can further convert it into fructose-6-phosphate. Both of these can enter glycolysis.

An Alternate Fate for Glucose—the Hexose Monophosphate Shunt

Unlike fatty acid synthesis, the Hexose Monophosphate Shunt (also called the Pentose Phosphate Pathway (PPP)) is considered to be an anabolic pathway—that is to say that we are constructing new molecules, rather than destroying them (Figure 7.1). In this pathway, Nicotinamide Adenine Dinucleotide Phosphate (NADP$^+$/ NADPH) and ribose 5-phosphate are produced. This pathway mainly operates within the cytosol of tissues that also synthesize fatty acids—namely the mammary glands, liver, and adipose tissue. But can also operate in other cell types, like red blood cells.

In the PPP, glucose-6-phosphate is converted to 6-phosphogluconlactone to start the process. The key enzyme is glucose-6-phosphate dehydrogenase (G6PD), which is absolutely required for the PPP to work. G6PD needs NADP$^+$ as a coenzyme and produces NADPH in the process[28] (Figure 7.14). The enzymatic conversion of glucose-6-phosphate to 6-phosphoglucolactone is an allosteric regulation point in which the concentration of the products and substrates for the reaction can change the enzymatic activity. In the case of the PPP, the substrate glucose-6-phosphate, and co-enzyme, NADP$^+$, drive the reaction forward. That is to say that during times of low energy demand, higher amounts of glucose-6-phosphate are being diverted to the PPP which increases the catalytic rate of G6PD. In addition, high amounts of NADP$^+$, which also occurs during low energy demand will drive the reaction. Conversely, high NADPH will allosterically inhibit G6PD enzymatic activity.

At the end of the oxidative phase of the PPP we have made ribulose-5-phosphate, which on its own doesn't do much, but can be converted into ribose-5-phosphate, an intermediate for nucleotide synthesis. Thus, this is one of the pathways that will not only produce reducing equivalents—NADPH, but also create substrates to make DNA and RNA[28]. If it is not needed for nucleotides, ribose-5-phosphate is converted into glycolytic substrates, namely glyceraldehyde 3-phosphate, and fructose-4-phosphate, which can be used in glycolysis. The enzyme performing this step is transketolase, which requires the vitamin thiamine (in a phosphorylated form) for activity.

Before leaving this pathway, let's talk a little more about the importance of the NADPH molecule. First, you should know that NADPH is one of the forms of niacin, or vitamin B3. Second, NADPH is key in helping to regenerate reduced glutathione, which is absolutely required for the scavenging of free radicals. In addition, NADPH is needed for folate metabolism, Vitamin D and other steroid hydroxylation and metabolism, nitric oxide synthesis, and immune function. Thus, as we divert glucose to this pathway, we are able to neutralize free radicals in a time when there may be a high proton gradient in the electron transport cycle, generating more free radicals. This occurs especially during low energy expenditure. Thus, it makes sense and is pretty nifty how our bodies divert the very thing that is in excess to fill a need that is produced by that excess! So, just because this is a "dumping" pathway, it isn't any less important than the more direct pathways that glucose normally takes. So, in summary, there are 3 major fates for glucose-6-phosphate: glycolysis, glycogenesis, or the PPP (see Figure 7.1).

Hexosamine Biosynthetic Pathway

The hexosamine biosynthetic pathway is known to be active in muscle, adipocytes, and pancreatic beta cells in response to nutrient availability. During low energy demand, about 2-5% of the glucose we take in is diverted to a pathway that is needed for hexosamine synthesis, especially when there is high glucose availability (refer back to Figure 7.1). Evidence suggests that this is also not just a "dumping" pathway, but actually a very responsive nutrient sensor, which acts at the transcriptional level to promote both glycolytic and lipogenic pathways[29]. Let's see how this pathway leads to nutrient sensing.

> **Bacteria have similar pathways**
>
> In bacteria, NAcGlc modifications are found in the cell walls. Some companies are using strategies to disrupt the hexosamine pathway in bacteria for drug treatments.

Just one step into glycolysis, fructose-6-phosphate can be funneled into the hexosamine biosynthetic pathway producing the end product uridine diphosphate N-Acetylglucosamine (UDP-GlcNAc) (Figure 7.15)[30]. This molecule is absolutely needed for post-translational modifications in making glycosaminoglycans, glycolipids, and secretory glycoproteins. Why? Because UDP-GlcNAc is used by the O-GlnNAc transferase (OGT) enzyme to add acetylglucosamine to serine and threonine residues of proteins (Figure 7.15). This addition modifies the activity of the protein or enzyme, usually leading to increased/decreased enzymatic activity or changes in protein stability and degradation. We'll talk about who these proteins are momentarily.

Getting back to the hexosamine biosynthetic pathway, glutamine fructose-6-phosphate aminotransferase (GFAT) (also called GlcN-6-P synthase) catalyzes the synthesis of glucosamine-6-phosphate from fructose-6-phosphate and glutamine, starting the hexosamine biosynthetic pathway. Fructose-6-phosphate levels are an allosteric activator of GFAT, while glutamine, which appears to bind after fructose-6-phosphate, is not[30]. The

> **Of mice and men:**
>
> Mice with a targeted deletion of OGT show a protection of diet-induced obesity—but with a consequence of having degraded muscle fibers and a reduced ability to move freely[31].

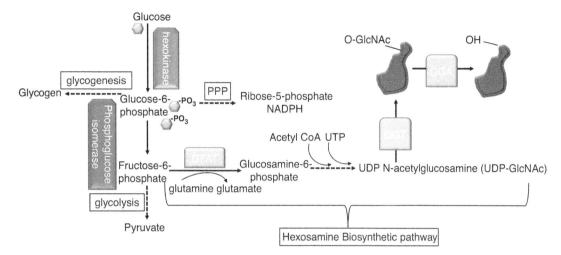

Figure 7.15: **Hexosamine Biosynthetic Pathway**. Interconnection between all of the fates for glucose and the hexamine biosynthetic pathway. G6P can be shuttled into glycogenesis and into the PPP, as alternatives to glycolysis. However, at the fructose-6-phosphate step, the choice is either for glycolysis or the hexosamine biosynthetic pathway. The enzyme glutamine fructose-6-phosphate aminotransferase (GFAT) produces glucosamine-6-phosphate from glutamine and fructose-6-phosphate. This enzyme is also called GlcN-6-P synthase. Adding acetyl CoA from fatty acid metabolism, and UTP from nucleotide metabolism, UDP N-acetylglucosamine (UDP GlcNAc) is produced from glucosamine-6-phosphate. UDP GlcNAc is used by *O*-GlcNAc-transferase (OGT) enzyme to add the O-GlcNAc to proteins, while O-GlcNAcase (OGA) removes the O-GlcNAc modification from proteins.

next steps involve the addition of an acetyl group from acetyl CoA (from fatty acid metabolism), followed by the addition of UDP, coming from uridine-triphosphate (as a result of nucleotide metabolism). This results in the formation of UDP-GlcNAc, which as mentioned above is the substrate for the OGT enzyme, leading to N-acetyl glycosylation of target proteins. The O-GlcNAc modification can also be removed from target proteins, again as part of a signaling nutrient-regulated pathway, through the action of an O-GlcNacase enzyme. The position of the O-GlcNac modification on a protein determines the downstream signaling pathways that the protein participates in.

One of the targets of OGT is the carbohydrate response element binding protein (ChREBP) which we discussed earlier in this chapter (see Figures 7.3 and 7.4)[29]. As you recall, ChREBP is post-translationally modulated in response to high glucose. When glucose is high and there is a low glucose need, protein phosphatase 2A dephosphorylates ChREBP, causing ChREBP to translocate to the nucleus and transcribe target genes. But that's not all. During this time, OGT targets ChREBP, placing an O-GlcNAc modification at serine #839 in the protein, increasing its ability to bind DNA, and therefore its transcriptional activity on target genes[29] (Figure 7.16). Overall, for this one transcription factor, changes in gene expression lead to increased glucose use, either as through glycolysis (by increasing gene expression pyruvate kinase for example) or as a result of diversion into *de novo* fatty acids synthesis (by increases gene expression of ACC). Of note, O-GlcNAc modification occurs on many different proteins, including histones that regulate how tightly DNA is wound, and while ChREBP serves as a model, one should consider many other points in nutrient sensing that could be affected by this pathway.

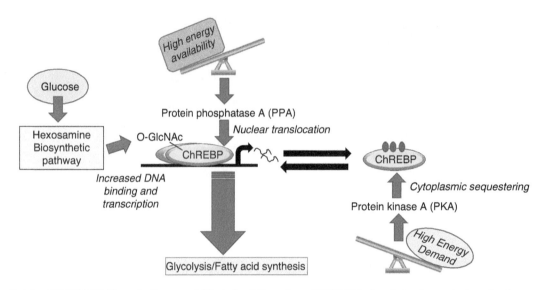

Figure 7.16: **ChREBP Regulation and Nutrient Sensing**. ChREBP (both isoforms) shuttles between the nucleus and the cytoplasm, due in part to phosphorylation on the transcription factor (keeping it cytoplasmic) or removal of the phosphate (translocating it to the nucleus). Glucose levels also increase the activity of ChREBP (alpha isoform only) through O-GlcNAc modification of the protein, which both increases its ability to bind DNA and increases its transcriptional activity. ChREBP target genes include those involved in glycolysis and fatty acid synthesis.

Summary

In summary, every time you eat a normal sized, 500–1000 calorie meal, around one-three hours after that meal, your metabolism is in a positive energy balance, and most of the processes discussed for carbohydrates are taking place. While some pathways will be ramped up, others will be turned down. Eventually though, storage will slow down, and use of stores will increase. All of this is normal. What isn't normal is the person who is chronically in the positive energy balance and is chronically activating these processes. In a later chapter, conditions of excess positive energy balance will be explored by building on this foundation of normal energy intake to discuss abnormal metabolic situations.

Points to ponder

- Try to diagram all pathways from glucose ingestion through storage or use, highlighting allosteric and covalent regulatory points in the pathways.
- Both metformin and resveratrol are AMPK activators[20]. Can you think about why this drug and this supplement might benefit diabetics?
- O-GlcNAc modification of ChREBP serves as a model of nutrient sensing by protein modification in response to high energy availability. Can you find other proteins that are modified by O-GlcNAc. What pathways are they in? How does modification affect their activities?

References

1. Xu X, So JS, Park JG, Lee AH. Transcriptional control of hepatic lipid metabolism by SREBP and ChREBP. *Semin Liver Dis.* 2013;33(4):301–311.
2. Sae-Lee C, Moolsuwan K, Chan L, Poungvarin N. ChREBP Regulates Itself and Metabolic Genes Implicated in Lipid Accumulation in beta-Cell Line. *PLoS One.* 2016;11(1):e0147411.
3. Iizuka K. The transcription factor carbohydrate-response element-binding protein (ChREBP): A possible link between metabolic disease and cancer. *Biochim Biophys Acta.* 2017;1863(2):474–485.
4. Shimomura I, Bashmakov Y, Ikemoto S, Horton JD, Brown MS, Goldstein JL. Insulin selectively increases SREBP-1c mRNA in the livers of rats with streptozotocin-induced diabetes. *Proc Natl Acad Sci U S A.* 1999;96(24):13656–13661.
5. Miao J, Haas JT, Manthena P, et al. Hepatic insulin receptor deficiency impairs the SREBP-2 response to feeding and statins. *J Lipid Res.* 2014;55(4):659–667.
6. Edwards PA, Kast HR, Anisfeld AM. BAREing it all: the adoption of LXR and FXR and their roles in lipid homeostasis. *J Lipid Res.* 2002;43(1):2–12.
7. Xu P, Zhai Y, Wang J. The Role of PPAR and Its Cross-Talk with CAR and LXR in Obesity and Atherosclerosis. *Int J Mol Sci.* 2018;19(4).
8. Kubota N, Terauchi Y, Miki H, et al. PPAR gamma mediates high-fat diet-induced adipocyte hypertrophy and insulin resistance. *Mol Cell.* 1999;4(4):597–609.
9. Witte N, Muenzner M, Rietscher J, et al. The Glucose Sensor ChREBP Links De Novo Lipogenesis to PPARgamma Activity and Adipocyte Differentiation. *Endocrinology.* 2015;156(11):4008–4019.
10. Martinez-Redondo V, Pettersson AT, Ruas JL. The hitchhiker's guide to PGC-1alpha isoform structure and biological functions. *Diabetologia.* 2015;58(9):1969–1977.
11. Nakamura MT, Yudell BE, Loor JJ. Regulation of energy metabolism by long-chain fatty acids. *Prog Lipid Res.* 2014;53:124–144.
12. Wilson JE. Isozymes of mammalian hexokinase: structure, subcellular localization and metabolic function. *J Exp Biol.* 2003;206(Pt 12):2049–2057.
13. De Backer I, Hussain SS, Bloom SR, Gardiner JV. Insights into the role of neuronal glucokinase. *Am J Physiol Endocrinol Metab.* 2016;311(1):E42–55.
14. Brouwers M, Jacobs C, Bast A, Stehouwer CDA, Schaper NC. Modulation of Glucokinase Regulatory Protein: A Double-Edged Sword? *Trends Mol Med.* 2015;21(10):583–594.
15. Lenzen S. A fresh view of glycolysis and glucokinase regulation: history and current status. *J Biol Chem.* 2014;289(18):12189–12194.
16. Hofmeister-Brix A, Kollmann K, Langer S, Schultz J, Lenzen S, Baltrusch S. Identification of the ubiquitin-like domain of midnolin as a new glucokinase interaction partner. *J Biol Chem.* 2013;288(50):35824–35839.
17. Han HS, Kang G, Kim JS, Choi BH, Koo SH. Regulation of glucose metabolism from a liver-centric perspective. *Exp Mol Med.* 2016;48:e218.
18. Marcelo KL, Means AR, York B. The Ca(2+)/Calmodulin/CaMKK2 Axis: Nature's Metabolic CaMshaft. *Trends Endocrinol Metab.* 2016;27(10):706–718.
19. Ozcan L, Wong CC, Li G, et al. Calcium signaling through CaMKII regulates hepatic glucose production in fasting and obesity. *Cell Metab.* 2012;15(5):739–751.
20. Mihaylova MM, Shaw RJ. The AMPK signalling pathway coordinates cell growth, autophagy and metabolism. *Nat Cell Biol.* 2011;13(9):1016–1023.

21. Hasenour CM, Wall ML, Ridley DE, et al. Correction: Liver AMP-Activated Protein Kinase Is Unnecessary for Gluconeogenesis but Protects Energy State during Nutrient Deprivation. *PLoS One.* 2017;12(8):e0183601.
22. Bidwell AJ. Chronic Fructose Ingestion as a Major Health Concern: Is a Sedentary Lifestyle Making It Worse? A Review. *Nutrients.* 2017;9(6).
23. Okar DA, Manzano A, Navarro-Sabate A, Riera L, Bartrons R, Lange AJ. PFK-2/FBPase-2: maker and breaker of the essential biofactor fructose-2,6-bisphosphate. *Trends Biochem Sci.* 2001;26(1):30–35.
24. Fenton AW, Tang Q. An activating interaction between the unphosphorylated n-terminus of human liver pyruvate kinase and the main body of the protein is interrupted by phosphorylation. *Biochemistry.* 2009;48(18):3816–3818.
25. Hilger C, van Hage M, Kuehn A. Diagnosis of Allergy to Mammals and Fish: Cross-Reactive vs. Specific Markers. *Curr Allergy Asthma Rep.* 2017;17(9):64.
26. Hu H, Juvekar A, Lyssiotis CA, et al. Phosphoinositide 3-Kinase Regulates Glycolysis through Mobilization of Aldolase from the Actin Cytoskeleton. *Cell.* 2016;164(3):433–446.
27. Meng X, Li M, Guo J, et al. Protein phosphatase 4 promotes hepatic lipogenesis through dephosphorylating acetylCoA carboxylase 1 on serine 79. *Mol Med Rep.* 2014;10(4):1959–1963.
28. Mullarky E, Cantley LC. Diverting Glycolysis to Combat Oxidative Stress. In: Nakao K, Minato N, Uemoto S, eds. *Innovative Medicine: Basic Research and Development.* Tokyo2015:3–23.
29. Benhamed F, Filhoulaud G, Caron S, Lefebvre P, Staels B, Postic C. O-GlcNAcylation Links ChREBP and FXR to Glucose-Sensing. *Front Endocrinol (Lausanne).* 2014;5:230.
30. Milewski S. Glucosamine-6-phosphate synthase--the multi-facets enzyme. *Biochim Biophys Acta.* 2002;1597(2):173–192.
31. Murata K, Morino K, Ida S, et al. Lack of O-GlcNAcylation enhances exercise-dependent glucose utilization potentially through AMP-activated protein kinase activation in skeletal muscle. *Biochem Biophys Res Commun.* 2018;495(2):2098–2104.

CHAPTER **8**

Fat Fates in the Fed State

In the one to three hours following a meal containing fats, the fats have been absorbed and then delivered to the tissues that require them, such as skeletal muscles, adipose, and other mitochondria-rich tissues. As discussed previously, this is done using chylomicrons, which package the fatty acids for transport and delivery (see chapter 6 if you need a refresher on this). As a reminder, in order to get the fatty acids from triglycerides into the tissues, the enzyme lipoprotein lipase cleaves fatty acids from triglycerides associated with the chylomicrons, and then the fatty acids can be taken up by facilitated transport by the transporters—Fatty Acid Translocase (FAT, also called CD36), Fatty Acid Binding Protein (FABP) and Long Chain Fatty Acid Transport Protein (FATP1) (refer back to Figure 6.11).

Triglyceride Synthesis

As also discussed briefly in Chapter 6, triglycerides are formed in the post-prandial state mainly in adipose tissue, but also to a minor extent in skeletal muscle, liver, heart, and pancreatic tissues. Whether they are synthesized *de novo* or come from the diet, the TAG synthesis mechanism is similar, just with different starting points. Let's look at fatty acids first. Following a meal containing fat, triglyceride synthesis will be favored as fatty acids are not the primary energy source being used. Likewise, if excess glucose is converted to glycerol-3-phosphate in adipocytes, triglyceride synthesis will be favored. Fatty acids are needed in the first and second steps of triglyceride formation, so let's talk about how these are used.

The first step for using fatty acids for either oxidation or for conversion to triglycerides is to convert the fatty acid to a fatty acyl CoA molecule (Figure 8.1). This process occurs via the enzyme acyl CoA synthetase—or rather a family of acyl CoA synthetase enzymes found localized to the endoplasmic reticulum (for use in triglyceride synthesis) or on the outer membrane of both mitochondria and peroxisomes (if converting to fatty acyl CoAs for oxidation). Note that this reaction requires one ATP molecule, but that the ATP is hydrolyzed to an AMP—effectively using two ATPs. Different isoforms of acyl CoA synthetase would perform the reaction at different locations—endoplasmic reticulum (ER) for triglyceride synthesis or the mitochondrial outer membrane for oxidation. There are actually four families of these synthetases and up to 25 of these enzymes in total, including—1. the very long-chain synthetases (ACSVL) (>21 carbon atoms), also known as fatty acid transport proteins (FATP), 2. the long-chain acyl-CoA synthetases (ACSL) (13–21 carbon atoms), 3. the medium-chain acyl-CoA synthetases (ACSM) (6–12 carbon atoms) and the 4. short-chain acyl-CoA synthetases (ACSS) (<6 carbon atoms), and within each of these groups there are several isoforms of each[1]. Note that FATP both transports long chain fatty acids from circulation into the cell and

Just peachy...or not!

According to genecards.org, mutations in the ACSL1 enzyme, which adds CoA to long chain fatty acids destined for beta oxidation can lead to an allergy to peaches and some other fruits—but it's not clear why!

can also add a CoA. The other members are found either on the ER or mitochondria, directing CoA addition to fatty acids for either triglyceride synthesis or beta-oxidation, respectively. As mitochondria preferentially use long-, and medium-chain fatty acids for beta oxidation, the ACSL and ACSM families are found mainly on the mitochondrial membrane[1]. The opposite reaction of removing the acyl CoA group can also occur, and this reaction is catalyzed by acyl CoA thioesterase (ACOT) enzymes (again a large family of enzyme isoforms) (Figure 8.1). However, while it appears that all of the ACOT enzymes have been identified, their role in fatty acid metabolism is less clear[2]. Most newer research, points to the fact that they may control fatty acid fate (i.e. oxidation versus storage) by allowing transport of fatty acids between organelles[2]. Stay tuned as more will likely be discovered about the ACOT enzyme family.

We've already gone over transport of fatty acyl CoA molecules into the mitochondria for beta-oxidation (see Chapter 4). In the fed state, especially when energy needs are low but energy availability is high, much of the fatty acids that are absorbed will be diverted to triacylglycerol (also known as triglycerides or TAG) synthesis. This process is also known as esterification of fatty acids, because of the ester bond that connects the fatty acids to the glycerol backbone. While the esterification process manly occurs in the adipose tissue, it is also occurring in liver, skeletal muscle, heart, and pancreas, and to be fair, any tissue with mitochondria and an endoplasmic reticulum has the ability to make TAGs.

For TAG synthesis, we have four steps to discuss (Figure 8.2). First, we start with glycerol-3-phosphate, and one fatty acyl CoA. In most tissues, glycerol is phosphorylated by glycerol kinase (GlyK) to produce glycerol-3-phosphate. In adipocytes, GlyK is not produced, and so glycerol-3-phosphate is produced by the enzyme glycerol-3-phosphate dehydrogenase (G3PD), which converts dihydroxyacetone phosphate to glycerol-3-phosphate. Note that in both reactions, energy is used—ATP in most tissues as the source of the phosphate group, and NADH in adipocytes, as the electron

> ### X marks the spot
>
> The gene encoding glycerol kinase is located on the X chromosome, but females (who have two X chromosomes) don't have a double dosage of the gene compared to males (who just have one X chromosome) due to X-chromosome inactivation.

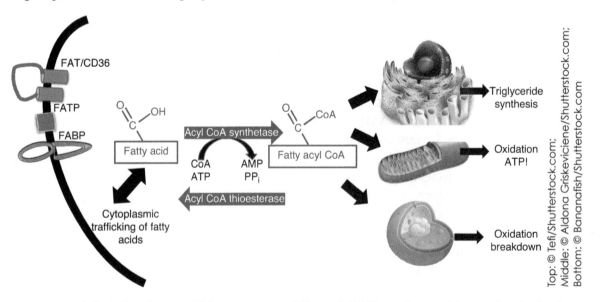

Top: © Tefi/Shutterstock.com;
Middle: © Aldona Griskeviciene/Shutterstock.com;
Bottom: © Bananafish/Shutterstock.com

Figure 8.1: Acyl CoA Synthetase, Thioesterase, and Fatty Acid Fate. Fatty acids are absorbed using CD36/FAT, FATP or FABP proteins on the cell surface, and are converted to a fatty acyl CoA using either ATP endogenous synthetase activity, or one of the other acyl CoA synthetases found on either mitochondria, endoplasmic reticulum, or peroxisomes. Acyl CoA thioesterases can remove the CoA and this allows for cytoplasmic trafficking of fatty acids.

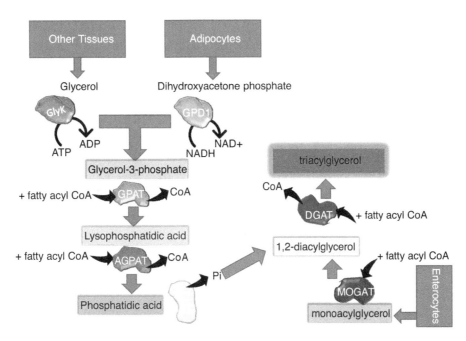

Figure 8.2: **Triglyceride Synthesis**. In most tissues, the starting material of glycerol, is phosphorylated to form glycerol-3-phosphate by the enzyme glycerol kinase (GlyK). Adipocytes don't have the GlyK enzyme, so they start with dihydroxyacetone phosphate and convert it to glycerol-3-phosphate using glycerol-3-phosphate dehydrogenase enzyme (GPD1). The reaction proceeds through glyceraldehyde-3 phosphate acetyltransferase (GPAT), and then 1-acylglycerol-3-phosphate O-acyltranstransferase (AGPAT), making phosphatidic acid, which can be converted to a 1,2,diacylglycerol by phosphatidic acid phosphatase (PAP), and finally to a TAG by diacylglycerol acetyltransferase enzyme (DGAT). In intestinal enterocytes, 1-monoacylglyceride can be directly converted to 1,2,-diacylglycerol by the enterocyte enzyme, monoacylglycerol O-acyltransferase (MOGAT).

donor in the dehydration reaction. Once the tissue has glycerol-3-phosphate, the reaction proceeds the same way in all tissues. First, through the action of glycerolphosphate acetyltransferase (GPAT), glycerol-3-phosphate is esterified with a fatty acyl CoA, producing lysophosphatidic acid and a leftover CoA moiety. 1-acylglycerol-3-phosphate O-acyltransferase (AGPAT), converts lysophosphatidic acid to phosphatidic acid by adding a second fatty acyl CoA, which can be converted to 1,2, diacylglycerol by phosphatidic acid phosphatase (PAP). In intestinal enterocytes, 1-monoacylglyceride can be directly converted to 1,2,-diacylglycerol by the enterocyte enzyme, monoacylglycerol O-acyltransferase (MOGAT). Finally, the enzyme diacylglycerol acyltransferase adds one more fatty acyl CoA, putting the third fatty acid onto the glycerol molecule and producing the TAG. All of these processes can occur in the endoplasmic reticulum (with the exception of G3PD enzyme in adipocytes, which is found in the cytoplasm). In most tissues, the first two steps in the process can also occur in the mitochondria. However, mitochondria do not have the last two enzymes in the process, so phosphatidic acid needs to migrate out of the mitochondria, to the endoplasmic reticulum to finish up the process of TAG synthesis. Remember that TAGs are usually stored in lipid droplets, along with cholesterol esters (which we'll discuss later in the chapter), and retinyl esters (derivatives of Vitamin A), surrounded by a phospholipid monolayer to contain it all.

One of the key questions about TAG synthesis is not how the TAGs are synthesized, but how the process is regulated. To date, the answer to this question is somewhat inconclusive but with several regulatory points in the pathway. The rate-limiting (and first) enzyme that is regulated is GPAT. Of the four GPAT isoforms, GPAT1 and 2 are co-localized to mitochondrial membranes, while GPAT3 and 4 are localized to ER membranes[3]. These localizations provide for unique and separate regulation for mitochondrial and ER-initiated TAG synthesis. Transcriptional regulation of the GPAT1 promoter has been well characterized and involves two transcription factors you should recognize—ChREBP and SREBP. As expected, signaling through glucose or insulin can activate the ChREBP transcription factor, and increase expression of GPAT1, whereas LXR interaction with the SREBP transcription factor enhances its binding to sterol regulatory sites in the GPAT1 promoter, also increasing transcription. (Remember that the LXR transcription factor also regulates the SREBP promoter). GPAT activity can also be increased post-transcriptionally, at the protein level through insulin signaling, and phosphorylation of serines and threonine residues, possibly through AKT[4]. Phosphorylation increases GPAT's enzymatic K_m[3]. Following a meal with lots of fat and/or carbohydrates, TAG synthesis is favored. Why? Because there is a naturally occurring rise in insulin, which will promote TAG synthesis and based on the information above—this can occur both transcriptionally and post-transcriptionally through GPAT synthesis and activation. Conversely, phosphorylation by AMPK decreases mitochondrial GPAT1, 3, and 4 enzyme activity[3]. When would we see AMPK activity in a cell? Yes—when energy levels are low, and when beta-oxidation of fats, rather than storage, should be stimulated.

Phospholipid synthesis

The phosphatidic acid phosphatase (PAP) enzyme is thought to be the rate-limiting enzyme for TAG synthesis within the ER—however, due to the difficulty in extricating these membrane-bound proteins from the membrane in order to study them, scientists have not yet gotten definitive answers to how, what, when, and where these enzymes might have allosteric or other regulators. What is known is that PAP, encoded by the *LIPIN1* gene is highly transcriptionally and post-transcriptionally regulated through multiple pathways[3]. In addition, phosphatidic acid, the product of that last mitochondrial-based reaction and the substrate for PAP has two pathways to choose from once produced. It can either migrate out of the mitochondria to continue in the TAG synthesis pathway, or it can be phosphorylated and then converted to become a phosphatidyl choline (Figure 8.3)[5]. Interestingly, this process involves use of cytosine triphosphate (CTP) as one of the starting materials to form the CDP-phosphorylated molecules for phospholipids[5]. While there are at least seven different phospholipids in the cell, phosphatidyl choline makes up the majority of these lipids. Choline is a vitamin-like substance which is found in many foods, but as it is the most abundant phospholipid, it can also be recycled during cellular recycling processes—hence it is not a vitamin and there is no recommended daily intake. Once it is conjugated to make CDP-choline, it is combined with diacylglycerol to produce phosphatidyl choline via the choline phosphotransferase (CHPT) enzyme (Figure 8.3). Thus, even if phosphatidic acid begins down the path towards TAG synthesis, it can still be diverted into phosphatidyl choline synthesis through this pathway. Another phospholipid, phosphatidyl inositol, is also synthesized from phosphatidic acid. Instead of forming 1,2 diacylglycerol via PAP, another enzyme, CDP-diacylglycerol synthase (CDP-DGS) acts on phosphatidic acid forming CDP-diacylglycerol (Figure 8.3). Notice that phosphatidyl inositol synthesis also uses a CTP! From there CDP-diacylglycerol is converted to phophatidyl inositol with the addition of the inositol head group via the phosphatidyl inositol synthase enzyme.

Here's where our understanding of the allosteric and covalent regulation of these processes end, at least for the purpose of this text—while phospholipids can regulate gene expression, especially through nuclear-receptor-type transcription factors[6], it is not clear if this is the mechanism of regulation for enzymes in these pathways, or if other covalent and/or allosteric regulation occurs to switch between phospholipid synthesis and TAG synthesis.

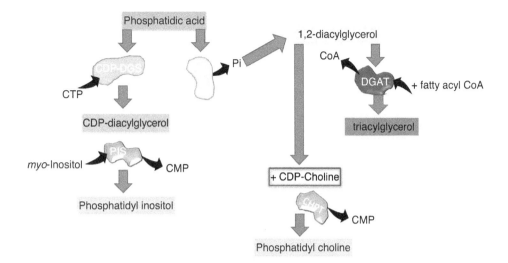

Figure 8.3: **Phospholipid Synthesis**. Phosphatidic acid has two pathways to choose from—either phospholipid synthesis or TAG synthesis. Likewise, diacylglycerol can either be converted to TAG or can be combined with CDP-choline by choline phosphotransferase (CHPT) to form phosphatidyl choline. The CDP moiety is formed from cytosine tri-phosphate (CTP), a pyrimidine nucleoside with three phosphates. Phosphatidyl inositol is produced from CDP-diacylglycerol by CDP-diacylglycerol synthase (CDP-DGS) and phosphatidylinositol synthase (PIS), respectively.

Cholesterol synthesis

Cholesterol is an important molecule composed of 27 carbons and 4 sterol rings (see chapter 4, as a reminder). Cholesterol esters have a fatty acid attached to the OH group and are more hydrophobic than cholesterol itself. Cholesterol is found in membranes as a buffer of sorts—increasing membrane fluidity at low temperatures and decreasing membrane fluidity at high temperatures. It is also an important substrate for steroid and bile-acid synthesis.

Did you know?

7-dehydrocholesterol (7-DHC) molecule is a precursor for *de novo* synthesis of Vitamin D which occurs in your skin through interaction of 7-DHC with UV light. So cholesterol isn't all bad—we need it to make our sunshine vitamin!

Cholesterol is found in animal products exclusively—most abundant in dairy, eggs, and meats (Figure 8.4). The average individual takes in ~400mg of cholesterol per day, with absorption of about 50% per day. This is higher than the recommendation by the American Heart Association of 300 mg a day. The rest of the cholesterol, as well as some endogenous cholesterol—up to 1 gram per day—is excreted. That means that the body needs to make about 800 mg (400 mg in diet *50% = 200 mg absorbed -1000 mg excreted) to maintain status quo. And in fact, when measured, the average person makes about 1000 mg of cholesterol per day. Is there a risk in eating too much cholesterol? That question is controversial, especially for those people who have high serum cholesterol levels—there are many articles both supporting low intake and debunking it (see for example a review by Dr. Maria Fernandez[7]). Since the human body can synthesize its own cholesterol, perhaps dietary cholesterol isn't what we should worry about, but instead worry about the things that provide the building blocks for cholesterol in our own bodies… Let's see how this endogenous synthesis happens.

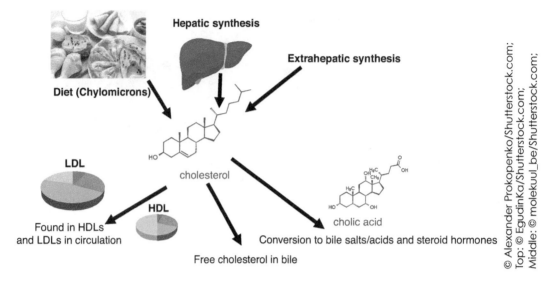

Figure 8.4: Cholesterol Synthesis, Storage and Use. Dietary cholesterol comes from animal sources only, and once absorbed it is incorporated into chylomicrons for transport to tissues. The liver, and tissues like the intestines, adrenal glands, and reproductive organs can synthesize cholesterol *de novo* starting with acetyl CoA. Cholesterol can be found circulating in the blood in lipoproteins such as HDL and LDL molecules, or can be secreted in the bile, either in free form, or converted into bile salts such as cholic acid. Cholesterol is also the building block to many steroid hormones. Green signifies cholesterol, yellow protein, blue TAGs, and orange phospholipids in the LDL and HDL diagrams.

Cholesterol synthesis occurs in the cytosol of cells, predominately liver cells—there are 31 steps needed for producing cholesterol, and 64 separate reactions—many of these requiring ATP and NADPH, making cholesterol is a highly energetically expensive process. While the starting substrate is acetyl CoA, and the ending product is cholesterol, we are going to skip going over the middle steps, except for one enzyme, HMG-CoA reductase, which is key in regulation of cholesterol production.

The first set of steps in cholesterol synthesis yield the molecule 3-hydroxy-3-methylglutaryl-CoA (HMG-CoA), which is formed from 18 acetyl CoA molecules (and using 18 ATPs, 14 NADPHs and 6 water molecules!). The next step, going from HMG-CoA to mevalonate is catalyzed by the enzyme HMG-CoA reductase. HMG-CoA reductase is allosterically inhibited by cellular cholesterol levels. This makes sense—right? If a cell has enough cholesterol, then there is no sense making more of that substance—especially since

> **Statins**
>
> One of the prescribed drugs on the market, statins, are actually inhibitors of HMG-CoA reductase. Brown and Goldstein won the Nobel prize for their discovery of HMG-CoA reductase and its inhibition by statins.

the process takes so much energy. HMG CoA reductase can also be regulated by covalent addition or removal of phosphate groups by kinases and phosphatases, respectively. When energy availability is high, such as after a meal, insulin will be secreted and will deactivate AMPK by activating a phosphatase that directly removes AMPK phosphorylation[8]. Since AMPK would normally work to phosphorylate HMG CoA reductase, inactivating it, this keeps HMG-CoA reductase active (unphosphorylated), by inhibiting the kinase that would deactivate it (Figure 8.5). Conversely, when insulin levels are low, AMPK would be active (and phosphorylated by kinases such as protein kinase C), phosphorylating HMG-CoA reductase, and rendering it inactive.

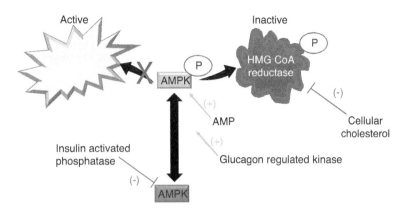

Figure 8.5: **Regulation of Cholesterol Synthesis**. The enzyme HMG-CoA reductase is inhibited allosterically by increased cellular cholesterol and covalently inactivated by phosphorylation, specifically by AMPK. AMPK can be activated by high cellular AMP levels and phosphorylation by a glucagon-regulated kinase and AMPK's activity is blocked by a phosphatase enzyme. HMG CoA Reductase is then active when there is lack of phosphorylation by AMPK, which would happen when insulin signaling is present.

Summary

As seen in this chapter, the liver plays a central role in the regulation of glucose and lipid fluxes during feeding. The coordinated control of carbohydrate and lipid fluxes based on nutrient availability are regulated by insulin and energy availability. TAG and cholesterol synthesis should be fine-tuned during normal energy flux, but as we will see in a later chapter, can become dysregulated when there are chronically high levels of energy (carbohydrates and lipids). Consider the roles of transcriptional and post-transcriptional regulation of the enzymatic processes as places where regulation can occur, or if lost, can become dysregulated.

Points to Ponder

➤ Consider the enzymatic synthesis of TAGs. Why would the pathway shuttle between the mitochondria and the ER? Are there advantages? Disadvantages? What about adipocytes whose process starts in the cytoplasm? How is this different from other tissues?

➤ Using Online Mendelian Inheritance in Man (omim.org) look up some of the enzymes in TAG synthesis. You will find interesting genetic lipid storage conditions. These conditions can provide information about the tissue-specificity of the various enzyme families.

➤ If the body can synthesize all the cholesterol it needs daily (needing ~800 mg, but synthesizing over 1000 mg daily), why would cholesterol be needed in the diet? Are vegans who eat little to no cholesterol healthier than non-vegans in terms of heart disease and obesity? Why or why not?

References

1. Steensels S, Ersoy BA. Fatty acid activation in thermogenic adipose tissue. *Biochim Biophys Acta.* 2018.
2. Tillander V, Alexson SEH, Cohen DE. Deactivating Fatty Acids: Acyl-CoA Thioesterase-Mediated Control of Lipid Metabolism. *Trends Endocrinol Metab.* 2017;28(7):473–484.

3. Wang H, Airola MV, Reue K. How lipid droplets "TAG" along: Glycerolipid synthetic enzymes and lipid storage. *Biochim Biophys Acta.* 2017;1862(10 Pt B):1131–1145.
4. Shan D, Li JL, Wu L, et al. GPAT3 and GPAT4 are regulated by insulin-stimulated phosphorylation and play distinct roles in adipogenesis. *J Lipid Res.* 2010;51(7):1971–1981.
5. Vance JE. Phospholipid synthesis and transport in mammalian cells. *Traffic.* 2015;16(1):1–18.
6. Crowder MK, Seacrist CD, Blind RD. Phospholipid regulation of the nuclear receptor superfamily. *Adv Biol Regul.* 2017;63:6–14.
7. Fernandez ML. Rethinking dietary cholesterol. *Curr Opin Clin Nutr Metab Care.* 2012;15(2):117–121.
8. Han JS, Sung JH, Lee SK. Inhibition of Cholesterol Synthesis in HepG2 Cells by GINST-Decreasing HMG-CoA Reductase Expression Via AMP-Activated Protein Kinase. *J Food Sci.* 2017;82(11):2700–2705.

CHAPTER 9

Protein Metabolism in the Fed state

All humans typically synthesize and degrade about 300 grams of protein per day. That's a lot (about 100 pennies which each weight about 3 grams, for comparison). In a normal balanced diet, the average human eats about 50 grams of total protein per day (RDA for protein is 0.8 grams per kilogram body weight[1]), and some of this can be broken down for amino acids. Other amino acids are obtained through endogenous (meaning inside the body) protein degradation—getting rid of the old proteins and using these to make new ones. We can get the building blocks for proteins from amino acid precursors—including histamine (makes histidine), and glutamate (makes glutamine) and alpha keto acids (makes alanine). Interestingly, the body uses about 25% of its ATP energy for protein catabolism daily[2]. Amino acids can also be used for energy production. However, different amino acids give different yields of ATP based on efficiency of the metabolic reactions, with methionine having the lowest efficiency at 28.6%, and glycine having the highest, at 68.9%. The efficiency of glycine as an energy source rivals glucose (70% efficiency) and palmitate (68% efficiency)[2].

The protein needs of the body, in terms of synthesis versus catabolism, determines the fates of amino acids. This is shown in Figure 9.1, which essentially summarizes the material in the chapter, showing all of the points that can be modulated in response to the state of the

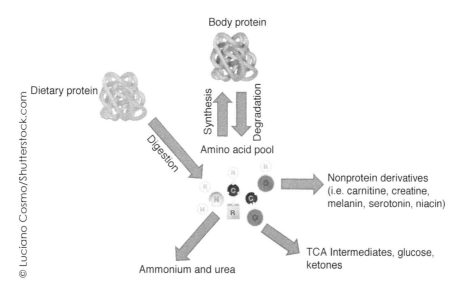

Figure 9.1: **Protein Fates**. Both endogenous (body) proteins, and dietary proteins can contribute to the amino acid pool. Amino acids can then be used for synthesis of new proteins, creation of non-protein derivatives, or their carbon backbones can be shuttled into the TCA cycle for energy production, while their nitrogen is disposed of as ammonium to make urea.

Table 9.1: **Amino Acids are Precursors to Non-protein Products.** Derived from the Food and Nutrition Board Dietary Reference Intakes for Macronutrients report. See text for citation information.

Amino Acid	Non-protein derived products
Tryptophan	Serotonin, Vitamin B3 (nicotinic acid)
Tyrosine	Catecholamines, Thyroid hormone, Melanin
Lysine	Carnitine
Cysteine	Taurine
Arginine	Nitric oxide
Glycine	Heme
Amino Acid Group	**Non-protein derived products**
Glycine, arginine, methionine	Creatine
Methionine, glycine, serine	Methyl metabolism
Glycine + taurine (from above)	Bile acids
Glutamate, cysteine, glycine	Glutathione
Glutamate, aspartate, glycine	Nucleic acids

body's needs. Of note, amino acids are not only used for protein synthesis or degradation—they are also the building blocks for many non-protein derivatives such as creatine (used to store phosphates to make ATP), carnitine (used in fatty acid transport, as we saw in Chapter 4), melanin (which is a skin pigment), and niacin (a B-vitamin that we can synthesize, but we still need to get in our diet) (Table 9.1)[1,3,4]. Note that many of the amino acids listed in this table are also essential amino acids (Table 5.1), which means that they are needed in our diets. We'll talk more about this later in the chapter. As we start to think about protein intake and use during the fed state, let's first remind ourselves about protein and amino acids in general.

> **Interesting fact!**
>
> Men can survive on a protein-free diet, but their sperm count drops by 90% after just 9 days[2].

A Review of Proteins and Amino Acids

There are 300 naturally-occurring amino acids in nature[2], and while humans only use 20 (23, if we count selenocysteine, selenomethionine, and pyrrolysine) of these for protein synthesis, others are present in the body and work in signaling pathways, including those directly impinging on cellular and whole-body metabolism[2]. In our bodies, skeletal muscle serves as the largest organ-based reservoir of proteins and amino acids, with up to 45% of the total protein mass of the body[2]. As we saw in chapter 5, each individual amino acid has its own unique characteristics (side chains) and metabolic pathways (deamination, transamination, and oxidation being the most common, but there are others[2]). Some amino acids are essential in our diet, meaning that we have to get them from foods, while others can be synthesized by our body's metabolic processes, and are considered non-essential from diet. However, just because an amino acid is non-essential for the diet doesn't mean we don't need it. There are many genetic conditions in which amino acid synthesis is impaired, and these can lead to devastating effects if not caught and treated by dietary supplementation or other interventions[5,6]. Likewise, inborn errors of metabolism that impair in amino acid breakdown can lead to the buildup of toxic substances such as ammonium ions, which can kill brain cells[2]. Even impairment of our "extra" amino acids—namely selenocysteine and selenomethionine can lead to myopathies, neurodegeneration, and cardiorespiratory failure[6].

Protein synthesis requires transcription of mRNA from the gene (DNA) that codes for it, splicing out of

introns (non-coding regions), and linking of the entire coding region of the mRNA, transport of the mRNA out of the nucleus to the rough endoplasmic reticulum or free ribosomes, translation of the mRNA by ribosomes, folding of the newly synthesized proteins, and modification of the proteins (such as glycosylation, phosphorylation, acetylation etc.). Finally, the protein has to be shuttled to areas where it is functionally needed. Each of these steps can be regulated, but we will mainly discuss the regulation of signaling cascades and degradation pathways in this chapter, as this is a major point of metabolic regulation of protein synthesis. In addition, note that protein synthesis rates are different for different tissue types (Figure 9.2)[7]. Remind yourself also of information in previous chapters where we discussed all of the post-translational modifications of enzymes that occur, specifically after insulin or glucagon stimulation.

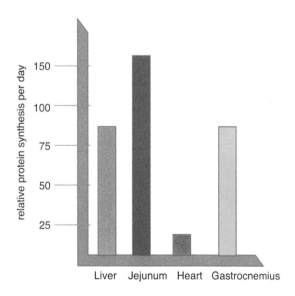

Figure 9.2: **Experimentally-derived Protein Synthesis Rates.** The figure was derived using Table 1 and with data from the article by Garlick et al., (1994)[7]. Two different methods for assessing protein degradation in rat tissues were used. As the raw data was not available, consider these values to be relative to one another, rather than absolute.

Recycling Old Proteins

There are two different pathways that can lead to protein degradation: The autophagy-lysosomal system and the ubiquitin-proteasome pathway (Figure 9.3). Proteins that are newly synthesized can be targeted directly for degradation, and this usually happens when the protein is misfolded, or perhaps cellular needs have changed and it is no longer needed. In addition, some proteins only have short "lifetimes" or in other words have a high turnover rate—because these proteins are often involved in very acute signaling pathways and act as a quick switch in cellular "states" that need to be flipped on and then turned off.

The autophagy-lysosomal pathways can target any protein but tend to work on larger protein complexes (Figure 9.3A). This system is also used to degrade long-lived highly stable individual proteins—especially structural proteins that are highly stable, but still need to be renewed periodically. Examples of these types of proteins include collagen and ferritin[8]. The autophagy-lysosomal system can also gobble up whole organelles for recycling! Once fused with a lysosome, the lysosomal hydrolases start to degrade proteins and other molecules. This entire system is regulated by energy availability, namely through the mTOR pathway[9].

The ubiquitin-proteasome pathway works to quickly remove small proteins and misfolded proteins. Ubiquitin is a small 8.5kDa protein that is made up of only 76 amino acids. The ubiquitin-proteasome process requires the use of ATP, during which ubiquitin is activated by the E1 activating protein, forming a bond between the terminal glycine amino acid in ubiquitin, and a cysteine residue in the active site of E1 (Figure 9.3B)[10]. Note that this reaction reduces ATP to AMP, so it is highly energetic. Ubiquitin is then transferred to a cysteine amino acid on E2 ubiquitin conjugating enzyme, and finally, using E3 ubiquitin ligase, it is transferred onto

Calorie restriction and lifespan

There is evidence from flatworms that the lifespan extension seen with calorie restriction is blocked if autophagy is blocked[11,12]. Researchers theorize that break down of proteins and cellular organelles is a necessary process to recycle amino acids and other cellular parts.

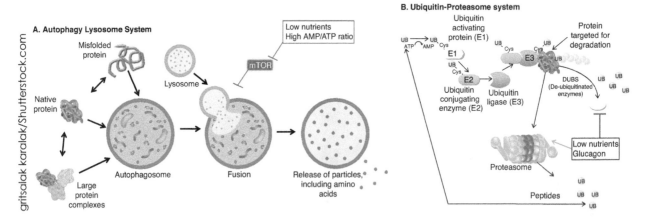

Figure 9.3: Protein Degradation Pathways. (A) Autophagy-lysosomal system. Native and misfolded proteins can be targeted to autophagosomes, but large protein complexes are usually always degraded there. Autophagy is blocked via the mTOR pathway which itself is turned off when nutrient or energy availability is low. **(B)** Ubiquitin-proteasome pathway. Ubiquitin activation requires ATP use, and several steps that result in conjugation of ubiquitin to targeted proteins, and proteasomal degradation. Ubiquitinated proteins are not always degraded, as de-ubiquitinating enzymes can also be activated. When nutrient or energy availability is low, proteasomal degradation is stimulated and de-ubiquitinating enzymes are inhibited.

the lysine amino acid of the targeted protein. This complex is then targeted by a proteasome—a very large, multi-subunit protein complex which subsequently degrades proteins into peptides for release and re-use. The ubiquitin can also be released and reused for ubiquitination of other proteins[10]. Note that low nutrient availability, and glucagon or epinephrine signaling through beta adrenergic receptors, can directly stimulate the proteosome to increase protein degradation. This all occurs through cAMP and PKA signaling pathways[12].

Anabolic Stimulation of Protein Synthesis

As food is taken into the body, glucose levels rise, and insulin is released. Among all of the other things that are stimulated in a fed state, protein synthesis is also stimulated. Insulin stimulates uptake of amino acids by individual cells, such as muscle cells, resulting in protein building. In addition, insulin reduces protein catabolizing events—which makes sense because in a fed state there are plenty of proteins and amino acids coming into the cells, so cells don't need to break down other proteins to release amino acids.

Insulin signaling is key to the anabolic response to feeding, and directly works by modulating mTOR (mechanistic target of rapamycin) activity (Figure 9.4). As we saw previously, inhibition of mTOR pathway increases protein degradation—so you might not be surprised to know that activation of the mTOR pathway increases protein synthesis. Insulin through the insulin receptor substrate 1 (IRS-1) signaling pathway can

> **What do you think?**
>
> If a high-protein meal results in amino acid uptake, but you need a glucose rise, followed by an insulin rise to maximally stimulate protein synthesis. If your meal is not mixed, i.e. a high carbohydrate-only meal or a protein-only meal, how do you get the protein-building effects?

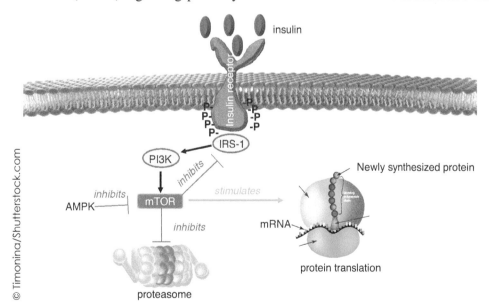

Figure 9.4: **Anabolic Regulation of Protein Synthesis and Degradation.** Insulin signaling activates IRS1 (insulin receptor substrate 1), which in tern activates PI3K (PI3 kinase), which activates mTOR (mechanistic target of rapamycin). mTOR signaling, through phosphorylation of ribosomal proteins leads to increased protein translation and decreased protein degradation. mTOR also negatively feeds back on IRS1. However, low nutrients or high AMP levels in the cell activate AMPK, which can phosphorylate mTOR, inactivating it.

directly activate the mTOR pathway. The net result is a decrease protein degradation and an increase in protein translation. The goal at the end of the day is to be in protein balance—having enough proteins to perform cellular functions, keeping these proteins in working condition, and having enough amino acids to make needed proteins in response to signals or any changes in the environment.

Essential Amino Acids

We can only synthesize new proteins if we have enough of the building blocks—namely the amino acids that make up the growing peptide chains. Even limiting one amino acid from the diet—and here we are talking about the essential amino acids which must come from dietary sources—will cause protein synthesis to come to a halt. Let's look at this more carefully.

Go back and take a look at Table 5.1. There are nine essential amino acids—tryptophan, methionine, leucine, isoleucine, lysine, phenylalanine, valine, threonine, and histidine. The level of essential amino acids in a diet affects how long, and at what level, protein synthesis occurs. This is especially true for leucine, glutamine, and arginine, which activate mTOR signaling when they are in sufficient quantities[13,14]. Of note, leucine is a member of the branched chain amino acids (which also include isoleucine and valine). Also, glutamine is a conditionally non-essential amino acid, which means that sometimes it is limiting and needed from the diet. As shown on Figure 9.5, activation of mTOR by leucine, glutamine, or arginine levels will decrease protein degradation pathways and increase protein synthesis pathways,

> **Malnutrition-a worldwide problem**
>
> Newer studies of childhood malnutrition consider inadequate protein intake, and reduced mTOR signaling as a direct cause in growth stunting in children until the age of 5 due to low circulating levels of amino acids[15].

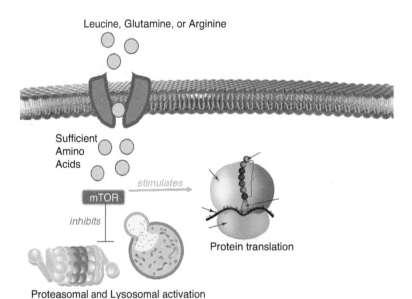

Figure 9.5: **Essential Amino Acid Regulation of Protein Metabolism.** Leucine, glutamine, and arginine, through their specific amino acid receptors can activate the mTOR pathway, leading to decreased proteasomal and lysosomal activation, and thus increased protein translation.

Table 9.2: **Food Sources of Complete and Incomplete Proteins, their Limiting Amino Acids, and their Digestion.** Examples of food sources are given, but the table is not meant to be comprehensive. Note that eggs are considered to have the best, and most comprehensive and dietarily available source of amino acids, when compared to other food sources. The bioavailability (BV) value is an estimation of the proteins absorbed from food that can be used by the body.

Food Source	Incomplete/complete	Limiting amino acids	BV Digestibility
Grains	Incomplete	Lysine, threonine, tryptophan	70–90%
Legumes	Incomplete	Methionine	70–90%
Soy	Complete	None	99%
Gelatin	Incomplete	Tryptophan	90–99%
Dairy proteins	Complete	None	90–99%
Animal and Fish meats	Complete	None	80–99%
Nuts	Incomplete	Lysine	~60%
Eggs	Complete	None	100%
Whey Protein Concentrate	Complete	None	100%
Casein	Complete	None	70–75%

similar to what we saw with insulin signaling[13]. Thus, once again, increased nutrient availability will lead to more proteins synthesized, and fewer degraded for "parts".

Individuals who have limited their intake of protein sources to those only from plant-based foods must be careful to combine sources so as not to limit one or more essential amino acids. As shown on Table 9.2, animal protein sources, including dairy, meats, and fish are generally "complete" proteins, meaning that none of the essential amino acids are missing in that protein source[4]. The exception is gelatin, which is missing the amino acid tryptophan. The only plant-based protein source that is complete is soy protein (although some sources claim that quinoa and chia seeds are also complete sources). All other plant-based sources of protein are considered "incomplete" protein sources.

Going nuts

Raw nuts contain phytates which can interfere with absorption of minerals like calcium.

Summary

Proteins are an essential macronutrient that are involved in both making functional enzymes and structural proteins for our physiological activities. When eaten, proteins provide the building blocks, namely amino acids, for synthesis of additional protein and non-protein molecules. When proteins are broken down to amino acids during digestion, the resultant amino acid pool in our bloodstream can not only be used for protein synthesis, but can also be used for oxidation as a non-carbohydrate or fatty acid source, and for synthesis of glucose, ketones, and fatty acids, as we saw in previous chapters. These amino acids also serve as signaling molecules to regulate whether individual cells will ramp up protein synthesis, or conversely, protein breakdown (Figure 9.6). The protein mTOR is key to this regulation. Both insulin and essential amino acid levels target mTOR activity. The net

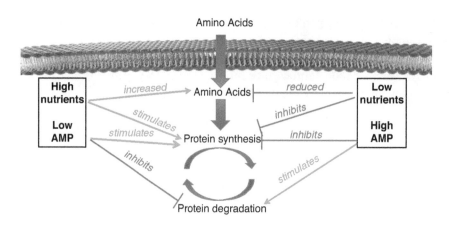

Figure 9.6: Nutrient Sensing and Protein Metabolism. A summary of the chapter is displayed. Remember that the turning on and off of mTOR is key to these signaling pathways (see previous Figures).

result is that protein degradation is high when energy (ATP/AMP) levels are low (high AMP), and protein synthesis pathways are high when energy (ATP/AMP) levels are high (high ATP).

Points to Ponder

➤ Individuals with sepsis due to infection, burns, tissue trauma, etc., show high rates of overall metabolism. What do you think this does to protein metabolism—would more proteins be synthesized or degraded? Why?

➤ Nuts have limiting amounts of lysine. Map out what would happen to someone on a diet of hazelnuts which actually are limiting for both lysine and methionine.

➤ Consider a person eating a high protein diet versus a high carbohydrate/low fat diet. What metabolic differences might one see for protein, carbohydrate, and fat metabolism?

References

1. Medicine Io. Dietary Reference Intakes: The Essential Guide to Nutrient Requirements. Washington DC: The National Academies Press; 2006.
2. Wu G. Amino acids: metabolism, functions, and nutrition. *Amino Acids.* 2009;37(1):1–17.
3. Engelking LR. Chapter 12 – Nonprotein Derivatives of Amino Acids. In: Engelking LR, ed. *Textbook of veterinary physiological chemistry.* Third Edition. ed. Amsterdam ; Boston: Academic Press/Elsevier; 2015:70–75.
4. Institute of Medicine (U.S.). Panel on Macronutrients., Institute of Medicine (U.S.). Standing Committee on the Scientific Evaluation of Dietary Reference Intakes. *Dietary reference intakes for energy, carbohydrate, fiber, fat, fatty acids, cholesterol, protein, and amino acids.* Washington, D.C.: National Academies Press; 2005.
5. de Koning TJ. Amino acid synthesis deficiencies. *J Inherit Metab Dis.* 2017;40(4):609–620.
6. Fradejas-Villar N. Consequences of mutations and inborn errors of selenoprotein biosynthesis and functions. *Free Radic Biol Med.* 2018.
7. Garlick PJ, McNurlan MA, Essen P, Wernerman J. Measurement of tissue protein synthesis rates in vivo: a critical analysis of contrasting methods. *Am J Physiol.* 1994;266(3 Pt 1):E287–297.
8. Wang DW, Peng ZJ, Ren GF, Wang GX. The different roles of selective autophagic protein degradation in mammalian cells. *Oncotarget.* 2015;6(35):37098–37116.

9. Glick D, Barth S, Macleod KF. Autophagy: cellular and molecular mechanisms. *J Pathol.* 2010;221(1):3–12.
10. Amm I, Sommer T, Wolf DH. Protein quality control and elimination of protein waste: the role of the ubiquitin-proteasome system. *Biochim Biophys Acta.* 2014;1843(1):182–196.
11. Morselli E, Maiuri MC, Markaki M, et al. Caloric restriction and resveratrol promote longevity through the Sirtuin-1-dependent induction of autophagy. *Cell Death Dis.* 2010;1:e10.
12. VerPlank JJS, Goldberg AL. Regulating protein breakdown through proteasome phosphorylation. *Biochem J.* 2017;474(19):3355–3371.
13. Broer S, Broer A. Amino acid homeostasis and signalling in mammalian cells and organisms. *Biochem J.* 2017;474(12):1935–1963.
14. Jewell JL, Kim YC, Russell RC, et al. Metabolism. Differential regulation of mTORC1 by leucine and glutamine. *Science.* 2015;347(6218):194–198.
15. Semba RD, Trehan I, Gonzalez-Freire M, et al. Perspective: The Potential Role of Essential Amino Acids and the Mechanistic Target of Rapamycin Complex 1 (mTORC1) Pathway in the Pathogenesis of Child Stunting. *Adv Nutr.* 2016;7(5):853–865.

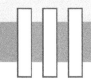

Energy Flux

CHAPTER 10

Fasting

Post-absorptive Period

What does Fasted Mean?

Is there is difference between the post-absorptive state and someone who is fasted (i.e. has not had a meal in a certain period of time)? People commonly use the word "fasted" to define the post-absorptive period, and we will use this term as well. However, in prolonged fasting (which for some people could be 12 hours, and others, depending on their habits, could be 24 hours) there are specific changes in metabolism, both hormonally and at the DNA/RNA level, to help the body to adapt to this situation. We will dive into prolonged-fasting and starvation at the end of this chapter.

It's Been 4–6 Hours Since Your Last Meal, What's Going On?

During the post-absorptive period, or fasted period (the time when macronutrients consumed in the meal have been digested, absorbed, and taken up by the body), what is happening? There are several conditions to be aware of in this post-absorptive period. Except for the liver, anabolic pathways have slowed or in some cases stopped, whereas catabolic pathways are now much more active due to high endogenous energy stores. Fatty acids have started to be the source for ATP production. Blood levels of glucose and amino acids have returned to pre-meal levels (i.e. they have lowered). In fact, glucose levels may dip below euglycemia, triggering the release of glucagon from the pancreas. Chylomicrons have been cleared by the liver and the TAGs that they were carrying are now stored in adipose tissue throughout the body. VLDL and LDL lipoproteins have become the most abundant lipoprotein types in the blood stream.

Blood Glucose Homeostasis

Glucagon

Whether we are in the post-absorptive state, or prolonged fasted state, the primary objective of the body is to keep blood glucose in homeostasis. The body wants to maintain a proper range of 5–7 mM or 90–126 mg/dL (euglycemia) of blood glucose. If we go above that (hyperglycemia) or below that (hypoglycemia), the body does what it can to return to euglycemia. This regulation is under control of two opposing hormones: insulin and glucagon. In a fed state, as mentioned earlier, insulin is released from beta cells in the pancreas in response to high blood glucose (see Ch. 6 for the mechanism of insulin release). In a fasted state when blood glucose drops below 5 mM, glucagon is released from alpha cells in the pancreas. Glucagon works to stimulate both gluconeogenesis (the making of new glucose) and glycogenolysis (the release of stored glucose from glycogen) in the liver, as well as lipolysis in the adipocytes. The liver then can release enough glucose to raise blood glucose levels back to euglycemia. If these pathways are unable to return blood glucose to normal, ketogenesis (the production of ketones) becomes vital to spare blood glucose for obligatory users. Ketones are also made in the liver from the building block—acetyl CoA, the product of fat oxidation.

> **Muscle glycogenolysis**
> Remember that the muscle can store and break down glycogen to form glucose. However, this glucose is never transported out of muscle, and instead is used locally. Glycogenolysis for producing circulating glucose always takes place in the liver.

Pancreatic Hormone Release

How does the pancreas know whether to release insulin or glucagon? If you remember, beta cells have the glucose transporter, GLUT2, which has a high Km for glucose (10–15 mM). On the other hand, alpha cells that secrete glucagon, have the glucose transporter, GLUT1, which has a low Km for glucose (5 mM) (Figure 10.1). Therefore, at high blood glucose levels, GLUT2 is transporting glucose into beta cells, stimulating insulin release and at low blood glucose levels, GLUT1 is

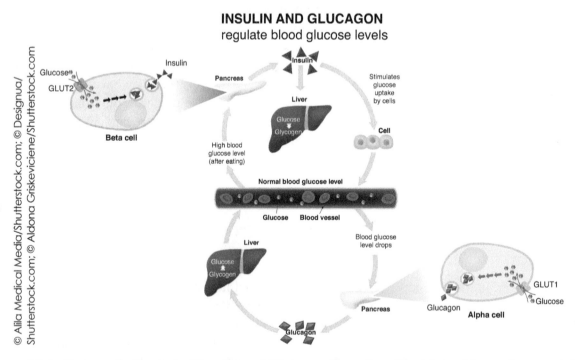

Figure 10.1: **Pancreatic Control of Insulin and Glucagon Secretion.** The islets of Langerhans contain islets with both alpha and beta cells. Beta cells have GLUT2 which respond to high glucose levels. Glucose uptake in beta cells causes release of insulin. Alpha cells have GLUT1 which respond to low levels of glucose and secrete glucagon.

Table 10.1: **Hormones Present in a Fasted State.**

Name	Location of Release	Stimulation for Release	Metabolic Function
Glucagon	Alpha cells of pancreas	Low blood glucose	Glycogenolysis, lipolysis, gluconeogenesis
Catecholamines (NE, E)	Adrenal medulla	Neural stimulation from the sympathetic nervous system	Glycogenolysis, lipolysis, gluconeogenesis
Cortisol	Adrenal cortex	Stress	Proteolysis

transporting glucose into alpha cells, stimulating glucagon release. The mechanism is similar for the release of insulin (refer back to **Figure 6.5**), as it is for glucagon. An increase of glucose uptake into the alpha cell, results in an increase in ATP production, which closes potassium channels, thereby depolarizing the cell. This change in voltage opens voltage-gated calcium channels, which allow for glucagon vesicles to dock with the plasma membrane, releasing glucagon into circulation. So, within the pancreas, two different cells types respond to two different levels of blood glucose, resulting in the release of glucagon when blood glucose levels drop, and insulin, when blood glucose levels rise.

Hormones

As shown in Table 10.1, we have several hormonal changes that occur during the fasted state (whether short-term or long-term). As mentioned above, when compared to the fed state, insulin levels are decreased, and glucagon levels are increased. In addition, catecholamines (norepinephrine (NE) and epinephrine (E)), may also be in circulation due to neural stimulation from the sympathetic nervous system. These hormones produced by the adrenal medulla, drive the same metabolic pathways as glucagon, mainly- glycogenolysis, lipolysis, and if needed gluconeogenesis. Another hormone cortisol, which is considered a stress hormone—is up, especially during a prolonged fast[1]. Cortisol, which is produced by the adrenal cortex, stimulates proteolysis or the breakdown of proteins.

Maintaining Blood Glucose

Glycogenolysis

Glycogenolysis, as you hopefully remember from our previous chapters, is the process of breaking down glycogen. This process occurs within skeletal muscle and the liver, although the purpose of the process in each tissue is different. In the skeletal muscle, the primary purpose is for local use, providing a source of glucose as a substrate for ATP synthesis. Muscle glycogen is primarily spared until times of stress or increased energy demand (i.e. exercise). On the other hand, in the liver, glycogen will be broken down to glucose, which will be released to maintain blood glucose levels. Glycogen is the "first line of defense" to maintain blood glucose, which as you should recall is a main goal for our body's physiology. As fasting continues, more and more glycogenolysis occurs—but this isn't a never-ending source. Depending on how active the individual is, and how high their stores are, the average glycogen stores will likely be depleted after 24 hours of fasting.

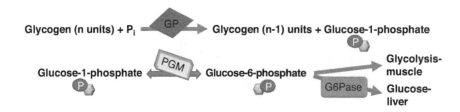

Figure 10.2: **Glycogenolysis and Glucose-6-Phosphate Production.** Glycogen phosphorylase (GP) acts on glycogen to cleave an alpha 1–4 bond producing glucose-1-phosphate. Phosphoglucomutase (PGM) converts glucose-1-phosphate into glucose-6-phosphate (G6P). In muscle, G6P enters glycolysis. In liver, G6P is dephosphorylated by glucose-6 phosphatase (G6Pase) and glucose is then secreted into blood circulation.

Glycogen Phosphorylase (GP)

The process of glycogenolysis requires the enzyme glycogen phosphorylase (GP) (Figure 10.2), which cleaves alpha 1–4 bonds from the non-reducing ends of glycogen, and adds phosphate group to glucose, creating glucose-1-phosphate. By looking at all the non-reducing ends that stick out of the glycogen molecule, you can clearly see how many spots there are for glycogen phosphorylase enzymes to release glucose easily and quickly, without disrupting the overall structure of the glycogen molecule (refer back to **Figure 7.7**).

Once we have glucose-1-phosphate, then phosphoglucomutase can move the glucose from carbon 1 to carbon 6, producing glucose-6-phosphate (G6P) (Figure 10.2). In skeletal muscle, G6P goes directly into glycolysis to produce ATP. In liver, G6P is dephosphorylated with the liver-specific enzyme glucose-6-phosphatase and becomes glucose, which can be secreted to increase blood glucose levels.

But where do glucagon and catecholamines come in? Hormones bind to G-coupled receptors on cells, which result in activation of rate-limiting enzymes that drive metabolic pathways in one direction. The rate-limiting step in this series of enzymes is GP. It is this first step where the cell 'decides' whether or not to break-down glycogen or not. In the case of glucagon and catecholamines, the G-coupled receptor activates adenylate cyclase, which converts ATP to cAMP, a potent intracellular messenger. cAMP activates protein kinase A (PKA)—part of the cellular signaling pathway which then phosphorylates glycogen phosphorylase kinase (GPK). GPK then phosphorylates glycogen phosphorylase (GP), making it active (Figure 10.3).

GP can also be allosterically negatively regulated by glucose. In the liver when glucose is high, it feeds back to negatively inhibit phosphorylated glycogen phosphorylase (GP-P) activity, by binding to another portion of GP-P, changing its shape. In the skeletal muscle, it is G6P that negatively allosterically regulates GP and GP-P. High levels on G6P, indicate adequate release of glucose, thereby slowing glycogenolysis. On the other hand, high levels of AMP and P_i, which would both be present in conditions of high energy demand (low ATP) serve as positive allosteric regulators of GP—AMP of the non-phosphorylated form (GP), and P_i of both GP and GP-P.

Another point of regulation of glycogen phosphorylase is through acetylation—the addition of an acetyl group to the protein. When would a person have high acetyl groups? What would this mean for energy demand? Does it make sense that glycogen phosphorylase would be regulated by acetylation? It does—because high acetyl groups would occur when we have a buildup of acetyl-CoA leading into the TCA cycle, or a buildup of acetyl CoA from beta oxidation. The acetylated

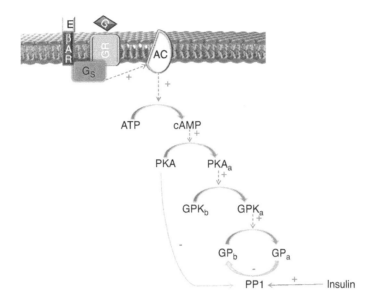

Figure 10.3: **Hormone Activation of Glycogen Phosphorylase (GP).** Epinephrine (E) binding to the (βAR) beta adrenergic receptor or glucagon (G) binding to the glucagon receptor (GR) activate a G-coupled protein that is stimulated (G_s), which activates adenylate cyclase (AC), which cleaves ATP to cyclic AMP (cAMP). cAMP activates protein kinase A (PKA), which phosphorylates the inactive glycogen phosphorylase kinase b (GPK_b) to the activate GPK_a. GPK_a phosphorylates the inactive glycogen phosphorylase (GP_b) to the active GP_a(GP-P), which now cleaves glycogen, releasing G1P. In the presence of insulin, insulin will activate protein phosphatase 1 (PP1), which dephosphorylates GP_a back to the inactive GP_b. PKA can phosphorylate PP1, decreasing its activity.

and phosphorylated glycogen phosphorylase "attracts" protein phosphatase 1 (PP1), which leads to de-phosphorylation and inactivation of GP. This means that GP's overall activity will be inhibited, and dephosphorylated when there are high acetyl groups present in the cells, leading to a decrease in glycogenolysis.

Glycogen Phosphorylase Kinase (GPK)

What about glycogen phosphorylase kinase (GPK)? This is also a place whether we can regulate GP because GPK is just upstream of GP, phosphorylating it (resulting in GP-P). GPK is made up of four protein subunits- alpha, beta, gamma, and delta. We can regulate GPK via phosphorylation (at the alpha and beta subunits), and by calcium binding (at the delta subunit, which is actually the familiar protein calmodulin). Each addition of either a phosphate or a calcium can make the enzyme active to phosphorylate GP (see Figure 10.4). The addition of both phosphates, and up to four calcium ions, is the most active form and results in high phosphorylation of GP. This ramps up glycogenolysis. As shown in Figure 10.3, glucagon stimulates the glucagon receptor, resulting in G-subunit activation and starting a cascade of kinases that lead to GP phosphorylation through GPK. At the same time, beta-adrenergic receptor activation by E can not only lead to PKA activation but can also lead to release of calcium from intracellular calcium stores via activation of the phosphoinositide cascade. Calcium, among many possible targets, will bind to GPK, further activating it. So, during these low glucose times, when beta adrenergic "fight or flight" (epinephrine) pathways are activated, we will get high GPK activation, and subsequently, high GP-P levels, and finally, glycogenolysis.

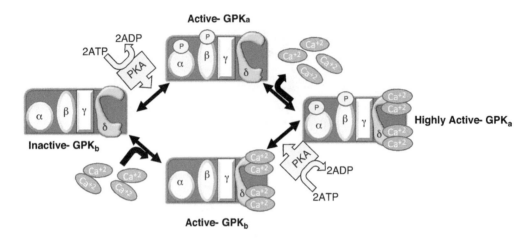

Figure 10.4: Glycogen Phosphorylase Kinase (GPK) Regulation. PKA can phosphorylate the alpha and beta subunits of GPK$_b$ making it active (GPK$_a$—GP-P). But GPK$_a$ can be more active when Ca^{2+} is bound to the delta subunit (calmodulin—CaM). Ca^{2+} comes from the sarcoplasmic reticulum in muscle or from endoplasmic reticulum in liver due to the activation of the phosphoinositide cascade. GPK is most active when bound by 4 Ca$^{2.}$. GPK can also have some activity in the GPK$_b$ form, when calcium is bound despite not being phosphorylated.

On the other hand, where there is available energy, the phosphate group can be removed from glycogen phosphorylase by PP1. This phosphatase is activated by insulin binding to the insulin receptor. This makes sense, when insulin levels are high, glucose levels are high too and we don't need to break down glycogen. Both liver and skeletal muscle "defend" the glycogen stores—in other words, maintain very tight regulation on muscle and liver glycogen levels, and immediately slow down and then stop glycogenolysis when the balance tips to a non-energy demanding state. As to not stimulate a futile cycle, PKA regulates PP1 through phosphorylation, inactivating it, so when glucagon and catecholamines are present, glycogenolysis will be active.

Fatty Acid Metabolism

FAs are the Major Substrate for Energy

During the fasted state, the primary substrate for ATP production are free fatty acids (FFAs) for all cells that have mitochondria (except for the brain, as FAs generally do not cross the blood-brain barrier). This is especially true for skeletal muscle, which is the primary site for FA oxidation during the fasting period. In addition, skeletal muscles store some intramuscular triglycerides (IMTGs). But where do tissues get additional fatty acids? As we saw in chapter 8, adipose tissue is the major site of TAG storage in the body. Through the process of lipolysis, TAGs are broken down in FFAs, which are released into circulation and bound to albumin for travel to tissues that can take them up and oxidize them. In addition, the liver is also releasing VLDLs into circulation, and these are packed full of TAGs that can be delivered to tissues via release by lipoprotein lipase, bound to endothelial cells of capillaries. However, compared to adipose tissue TAG release, VLDLs play a minor role in providing FFAs to active cells.

Lipolysis

Your body is designed to use fats for energy, and in fact there's a lot of energy in fat, so it makes sense. However, FFA oxidation uses more oxygen than glucose oxidation in the ETC; consequently, this can be rate-limiting because fat oxidation isn't as fast. So, when you need quick energy, look to glucose. For long-lasting energy,

look to fats. As mentioned earlier, fatty acids are the predominant substrate for ATP production in cells (like skeletal muscle, and liver, and skin) that have mitochondria, in the fasted state. This is really important in the liver and in skeletal muscle, because it allows for the preservation of glycogen stores. In the liver, there is a constant need for ATP, and so stored FFAs in the liver or surrounding the liver, can serve as a source of substrate for ATP production.

Lipolysis is the process of breaking down TAGs to liberate fatty acids, primarily in adipose tissue through hydrolysis. This happens sequentially, with each TAG becoming a diacylglycerol (DAG) plus a fatty acid, and then the DAG becoming a monoacylglycerol (MAG) plus a fatty acid, and finally the MAG becoming a glycerol and a fatty acid. All of these reactions happen through specific enzymes (Figure 10.5), in sequence: adipose triacylglycerol lipase (ATGL), followed by hormone sensitive lipase (HSL) and monoglyceride lipase (MGL). Perilipin A and CGI-58 are regulatory proteins. Perilipin A is thought to bind to the fat droplet preventing lipases from acting on the TAGs. CG-158 is known to bind to perilipin A, playing a role on its binding to the fat droplet. Lipolysis is tightly regulated and is favored in a fasted state, a low-carbohydrate diet, low-intensity exercise, and post-exercise recovery, as the provider of FAs for beta oxidation and ATP production.

As mentioned, lipolysis is tightly regulated. It can be activated by glucagon or catecholamines—which makes sense, since these are high when in a fasted state. Within adipocytes, there is a constant low-level activity of ATGL, providing enough FFAs for adipose tissue needs. During a fasted state, lipolysis is what we call "stimulated." Stimulated lipolysis is needed to break down fats and provide free fatty acids for other tissues to use for energy. Conversely, lipolysis is inhibited by insulin, as insulin levels would be high when we are in a fed state.

Let's use glucagon-stimulated lipolysis as an example of the signaling pathway. Glucagon binds to the glucagon receptor, which is a G-coupled protein, that stimulates adenylate cyclase to covert ATP to cAMP. cAMP starts the signaling cascade by activating Protein kinase A (PKA). PKA is a kinase and therefore phosphorylates CGI-58, perilipin A, ATGL, and HSL (note that MGL is not a

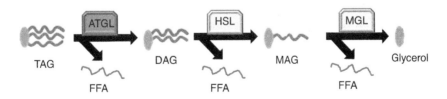

Figure 10.5: **Enzymatic Pathway for Lipolysis.** Triglycerides (TAGs) are hydrolyzed to diglycerides (DAGs) and a free fatty acid (FFA) by the enzyme adipose triglyceride lipase (ATGL) primarily with a minor contribution by hormone sensitive lipase (HSL). DAGs are hydrolyzed to monoglycerides (MAGs) and a FFA by HSL. MAGs are hydrolyzed to a FFA and a glycerol molecule (G) by monoglyceride lipase (MGL).

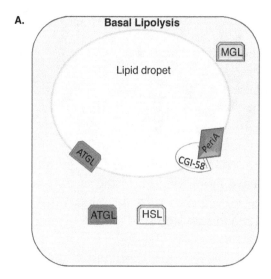 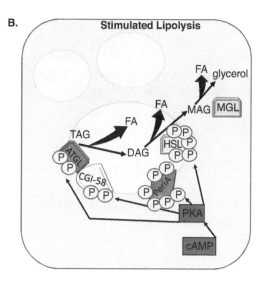

Figure 10.6: **Basal and Stimulated Lipolysis.** (**A**) During basal lipolysis, the lipases and regulatory proteins are dephosphorylated. CGI-58 is bound in perilipin. Adipose triglyceride lipase (ATGL) is slightly active providing small amounts of free fatty acids (FFAs) to adipocytes. (**B**) When the lipolysis pathway is turned on, protein kinase A (PKA) phosphorylates ATGL, CGI-58, perilipin A, and HSL. Phosphorylated perilipin A is now inactive and phosphorylated CGI-58 now binds to ATGL, increasing its activity. Phosphorylation of ATGL and HSL make these lipases fully active driving lipolysis.

target of PKA and is active even in a non-phosphorylated state) (Figure 10.6). Remember, phosphorylation is an example of covalent modification of an enzyme. When perilipin is phosphorylated, it causes the release of CGI-58 and perilipin A also moves out of the way. Phosphorylated CGI-58 then attaches to ATGL, increasing ATGL's enzymatic activity. The phosphorylation of ATGL and HSL turns these lipases on, leading to hydrolysis of the TAG.

Adipocytes have a glucagon receptor, and both beta- and alpha-adrenergic receptors, which can bind epinephrine and norepinephrine. When the alpha (α_2) receptor is stimulated, an inhibitory G-protein is activated, which can decrease lipolysis. Adipocytes and other cells have different ratios of beta- and alpha-adrenergic receptors. This helps to balance the metabolic response to norepinephrine and epinephrine so that the process can easily be toned down or turned up, depending on the ratio of those receptors. Insulin receptors are also on the adipocyte. Insulin blocks the signaling pathway for lipolysis by activating phosphodiesterase (PDE) and protein phosphatase 2 (PP2). PDE converts cAMP into AMP, removing the intracellular messenger and turning off the signaling cascade. PP2 dephosphorylates CGI-58, perilipin A, ATGL, and HSL, thereby turning off lipolysis (see Figure 10.7).

Lipolysis is also regulated allosterically. FAs allosterically inhibit lipolysis—why? Because if there are already a lot of fatty acids floating around, then you don't want to release more. Only the HSL enzyme is inhibited allosterically, which means that only the production of MAGs are blocked. What this means for the process is that DAGs could still be made even when there are high levels of fatty acids. However, the cell is smart, and because DAGs can be used for cell membrane components, they are often needed by cells even when energy isn't.

The products of lipolysis are 3 FFAs and a glycerol molecule. FAs are released by the adipocyte and are bound to albumin in the blood. They are then circulated to cells/tissues that need them. Glycerol is also released and can be used for gluconeogenesis in the liver or can be phosphorylated

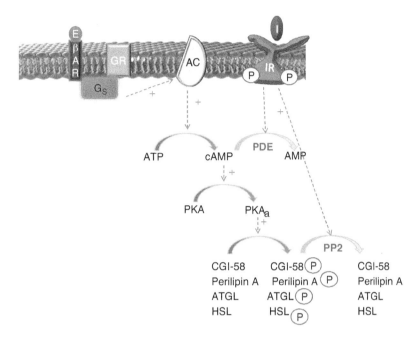

Figure 10.7: **Insulin-Mediated Inhibition of Lipolysis.** When insulin (I) binds to the insulin receptor (IR), it activates phosphodiesterase (PDE), which converts cAMP to AMP; and activates protein phosphatase 2 (PP2), which dephosphorylates CGI-58, perilipin, ATGL, and HSL, ending stimulated lipolysis.

to glycerol-3-phosphate by glycerol kinase, which is the form needed for TAG synthesis (although this doesn't happen in the fasted state). So, both products are useful—let's take a look at these in more detail.

Fatty Acid Uptake

In the fasted state, your liver and skeletal muscles are actively oxidizing FAs to produce energy. Short and medium chain fatty acids can get into the cell and mitochondria directly, without going through a transport step. However, the long chain FAs must be transported into the cell using a fatty acid transporter. Using facilitated diffusion, one of the following FA transporters: FABP, FATP4, or FAT/CD36, can uptake the FFA into the cell (see chapter 6). To use the FFA, a CoA needs to be attached using fatty acyl CoA synthetase. This process uses the equivalent of 2 ATPs converting ATP into AMP.

Fatty Acid Transport into the Mitochondria

For FFAs to be transported into the mitochondria, they must be attached to a carnitine molecule. The fatty acyl CoA is acted on by carnitine palmitoyl transferase 1 (CPT1) (also known as carnitine acyl transferase 1 (CAT1), which removes the CoA and adds the carnitine moiety making a fatty acyl carnitine molecule. Carnitine acyl transferase then transfers the fatty acid across the membrane, where carnitine palmitoyl transferase 2 (CPT2) (or CAT2) removes the carnitine moiety and adds back the CoA (see chapter 4). It was recently discovered that the fatty acid transporter FAT/CD36 is also located on the mitochondrial membrane and works with the carnitine shuttle system. Once the fatty acyl CoA is in the mitochondria, beta oxidation can begin.

Beta-oxidation of Fatty Acids

Regulation

Beta oxidation is the process by which fatty acids are cleaved two carbons at a time to make an acetyl CoA. So, for a 16-carbon fatty acid, you would get 8 acetyl CoA molecules (see chapter 4 and figure 4.9). There is no single enzymatic reaction in the beta oxidation pathway that is rate limiting, so if fatty acyl CoAs are provided, they will be oxidized. Therefore, beta oxidation is regulated by limiting fatty acid entry into mitochondria by the carnitine shuttle system, specifically by CPT1.

Malonyl-CoA is a potent inhibitor of CPT1, which prevents entry of fatty acids into the mitochondria. Where do we get malonyl CoA? There are two key enzyme isoforms that produce malonyl CoA—acetyl CoA carboxylase (ACC), in the forms ACC1 and ACC2. ACC1 makes malonyl-CoA in the liver and adipose tissue as part of FA synthesis for TAG storage, whereas ACC2 makes malonyl CoA mostly in skeletal muscle as a regulator of beta oxidation. We've seen this before, so make sure you go back and look at beta oxidation in chapter 4. ACC produces malonyl CoA from an acetyl CoA and a bicarbonate molecule; this reaction is regulated. In the fasting state, this enzyme will be inhibited through the activity of AMPK (see Figure 10.8). Remember that in a fasting state, generally phosphorylation activates enzymes, but in this case, AMPK inhibits ACC and activates another enzyme, malonyl CoA decarboxylase (MCD), which can convert malonyl CoA back to acetyl CoA. In addition, with the removal of malonyl CoA, CPT1 is now active again, allowing for fatty acyl CoA entry into the mitochondria. Remember that AMPK is active in times of energy demand so it makes sense that AMPK is going to be active when we need to have available acetyl CoA for making ATP. Citrate is an allosteric activator of ACC, indicating that energy is in abundance, whereas palmitoyl CoA and AMP are negative allosteric inhibitors, indicating that there is an energy need, allowing for acetyl CoA to be produced.

Prolonged Fast

Gluconeogenesis

During a prolonged fast (12- 20 or more hours), glycogen stores in the liver that maintain blood glucose, may begin to be depleted. To be able to maintain euglycemia, the liver (and to a small

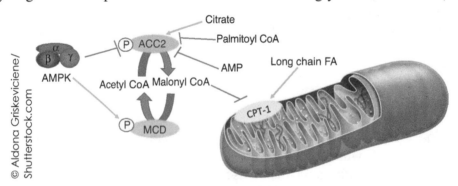

Figure 10.8: **Regulation of Carnitine Palmitoyl Transferase (CPT1) by Malonyl CoA.** Malonyl CoA levels allosterically inhibit CPT1, blocking fatty acid entry into the mitochondria. Both acetyl CoA carboxylase 1 and 2 (ACC 1/2), produce malonyl CoA, but it is ACC2 that is found in skeletal muscle and leads to the production of malonyl CoA that blocks CPT1. Malonyl CoA decarboxylase (MCD) removes malonyl CoA, producing acetyl CoA. ACC 1/2 and MCD are regulated by adeonosine monophosphate kinase (AMPK), which is active in times of energy demand. AMPK phosphorylates both ACC 1/2 and MCD, making ACC 1/2 inactive and MCD active. Citrate allosterically activates ACC and palmitoyl CoA and AMP allosterically inhibit ACC.

extent, the kidney) needs to make glucose. This process of making glucose is called gluconeogenesis. Gluconeogenesis is essentially glycolysis in reverse! In gluconeogenesis, glucose is synthesized from non-carbohydrate precursors such as glycerol, lactate, pyruvate, and the carbon skeletons of amino acids. You might not realize this, but 10% of gluconeogenesis actually takes place in the kidney. As we learn more about the organ, we find out that it is not all about waste, but actually maintains blood mineral homeostasis, produces the active form of Vitamin D- calcitriol, and as we just found out, the kidney can also make glucose! This makes a lot of sense as some of the "waste" products of lactate, glycerol, pyruvate and amino acids are flowing around in the blood and can easily be filtered out when needed by the kidney. However, the main location for gluconeogenesis is the liver, where approximately 90% of new glucose synthesis takes place.

The process is relatively simple as glycolysis goes in reverse with a few exceptions. Three key reactions in glycolysis run by glucokinase, PFK1, and pyruvate kinase (which as you might recall are regulated steps in glycolysis, and not reversible) are replaced by reactions involving the enzymes pyruvate carboxylase, phosphoenolpyruvate carboxykinase (PEPCK), fructose-1, 6 bisphosphatase and glucose-6-phosphatase (Figure 10.9). Gluconeogenesis begins with glucogenic precursors like lactate, glycerol, and amino acids (specifically alanine) being converted into pyruvate or other intermediates and entering the gluconeogenesis pathway. Starting with pyruvate and to bypass pyruvate kinase, two enzymatic reactions take place. Pyruvate and a bicarbonate ion are converted to oxaloacetate by pyruvate carboxylase. The oxaloacetate is converted to phosphoenolpyruvate by phosphoenolpyruvate

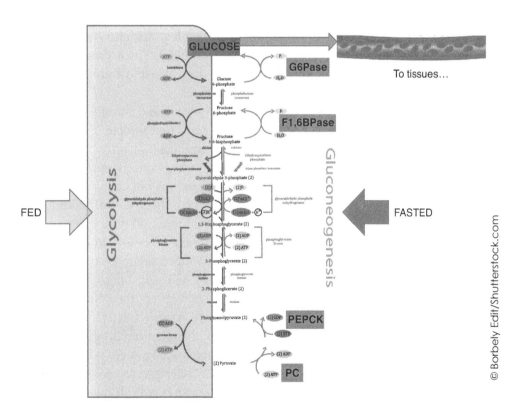

Figure 10.9: **The Process of Gluconeogenesis.** Gluconeogenesis occurs in the liver and to a small extent in the kidney under fasting conditions. Glucogenic precursors are converted into pyruvate, which sends glycolysis in reverse. Pyruvate carboxylase (PC) and phsophoenolpyruvate carboxykinase (PEPCK) bypass the non-reversible enzymatic reaction of pyruvate kinase. Fructose 1,6 bisphosphatase (F16BPase) bypasses the non-reversible reaction of phosphofructokinsae 1 (PFK1). Glucose-6 phosphatase (G6Pase) bypasses the non-reversible reaction of glucokinase, thereby producing glucose, which can be released to the bloodstream.

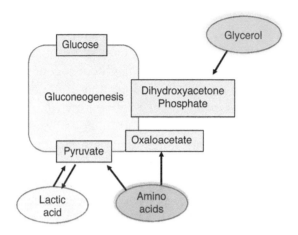

Figure 10.10: **Glucogenic Precursors entering Gluconeogenesis.** Glycerol picked up by the liver as a result of lipolysis in adipose and other tissues, is converted to dihydroxyacetone phosphate (DHAP) and then enters the gluconeogenesis pathway. Lactate is converted to pyruvate by lactate dehydrogenase (LDH) and then enters the gluconeogenesis pathway. Amino acids (specifically alanine) can be converted to pyruvate or oxaloacetate and enter the gluconeogenesis pathway at that point.

carboxykinase (PEPCK) using a GTP. The process then proceeds backwards through all the enzymes that are reversible, until it gets to fructose 1,6, biphosphate, where fructose 1, 6, bisphosphate is hydrolyzed into fructose-6-phosphate using fructose 1,6 bisphasphotase (F1,6BPase), bypassing phosphofructokinase 1 (PFK1). One step later we have glucose-6-phosphate which is hydrolyzed into glucose by glucose-6-phosphatase (G6Pase), bypassing glucokinase. For both of these reactions, instead of using ATP as they do in the forward (glycolysis) reaction, they cleave off an inorganic phosphorous, which could be used to make additional ATPs in other reactions.

As the body starts to breakdown fats and proteins, glycerol and amino acids, or lactate from anaerobic glycolysis are produced. These substrates can enter the gluconeogenesis pathway as the points indicated (Figure 10.10). Glycerol can enter gluconeogenesis as dihydroxyacetone phosphate (DHAP) through two enzymatic reactions using glycerol kinase and glycerol phosphate dehydrogenase. Amino acids can be converted to either pyruvate or oxaloacetate and enter the gluconeogenesis pathway. Alanine is the primary amino acid used by the liver to make glucose. Alanine transaminase (ALT) converts pyruvate to alanine in a coupled reaction where branch chained amino acids (BCAAs) are catabolized to glutamate during proteolysis. To continue BCAA catabolism, the conversion of pyruvate to alanine is favored because it produced alpha keto glutarate which is the needed substrate for branched chain aminotransferase (BCAT), see Figure 12.6. Alanine is then picked up by the liver and converted to pyruvate, which then enters the gluconeogenesis pathway (Figure 10.11). ALT is transcriptionally increased with exercise[2]. Lastly, lactate, the product of anaerobic metabolism can also be converted to pyruvate by lactate dehydrogenase (LDH) and enter gluconeogenesis. Anytime glycolysis, aerobic or anaerobic, is active there will be some lactate produced. The Cori cycle illustrates this process—working muscle produces lactate, which is picked up by the liver and converted to glucose through gluconeogenesis, which release glucose into circulation, whereby working muscle then picks the glucose back up and oxidizes it through glycolysis (Figure 10.11). In addition, three substrates of the TCA cycle: succinyl CoA, fumarate, and alpha ketoglutarate can all enter gluconeogenesis by being converted into oxaloacetate.

So, where are the gluconeogenesis allosteric regulation points? The first one is pyruvate carboxylase, which is allosterically activated by high acetyl CoA levels. Fatty acid oxidation spares blood glucose. So,

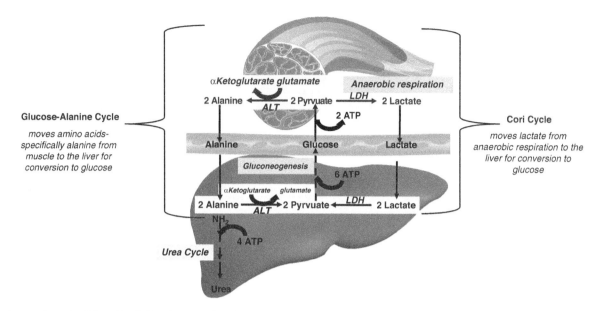

Figure 10.11: **The Cori Cycle and the Glucose-Alanine Cycle.** In the Glucose-alanine cycle, working muscle goes through proteolysis producing amino acids. Alanine, specifically, is released and taken up by the liver. Alanine transaminase (ALT) converts alanine to pyruvate, which enters gluconeogenesis. At the same time in the Cori cycle, working muscle is producing lactate via anaerobic glycolysis. Lactate is also released and picked up by the liver. Lactate is converted to pyruvate via lactate dehydrogenase (LDH), which enters gluconeogenesis. The glucose that is produced by either the glucose-alanine cycle or the Cori cycle is then released into circulation, where working muscle can take it up and continue ATP formation. Other amino acids can be used for gluconeogenesis. Deamination of these amino acids in the liver produces ammonium ions, which enter into the urea cycle.

with high levels of FA oxidation in the liver, high levels of acetyl CoA will be produced, signaling a need to make glucose. The second one is fructose- 1,6 bisphosphatase, which allosterically inhibited by rising AMP levels, signaling an energy deficit. Secondly, insulin (present in a fed state), can lead to the production of fructose 2,6 bisphosphate, by activating PFK2, an alternative form of PFK1[3]. PFK2 is active when dephosphorylated, so in the presence of insulin which activates protein phosphatases, PFK2 will be active, producing fructose 2,6 bisphosphate, which inhibits 1,6- bisphosphatase, blocking gluconeogenesis.

As mentioned earlier in chapter 3, glycolysis is also regulated allosterically and some of the same allosteric regulators that stimulate or block gluconeogenesis can at the same time stimulate or block glycolysis, so that only one pathway is active at time. So not only does fructose 2,6 bisphosphate inhibit 1,6- bisphosphatase, fructose 2,6 bisphosphate also, allosterically activates PFK1[4], driving glycolysis. Remember, PFK1 is also allosterically activated by AMP and ADP (AMP is also an inhibitor of 1,6- bisphosphatase); and PFK1 is inhibited allosterically by ATP and citrate. Lastly, pyruvate kinase is allosterically inhibited by ATP, slowing glycolysis and allosterically activated by fructose 1,6 bisphosphate, the product of PFK1, increasing glycolytic flux.

Well then, where does PFK2 come in in a fasted state? When glucagon is present, it activates PKA, which phosphorylates PFK2, thereby inhibiting it. So, in a fasted state, PFK2 will not produce the potent allosteric inhibitor, fructose 2,6 bisphosphate, of fructose 1,6- bisphosphatase, thereby allowing gluconeogenesis to proceed.

Not only does insulin activate protein phosphatases, it also drives transcription of glycolysis enzymes and blocks transcription of gluconeogenesis enzymes. The presence of insulin increases the transcription of glucokinase[5], PFK1[6], and pyruvate kinase[5]—all of which drive glycolysis. The

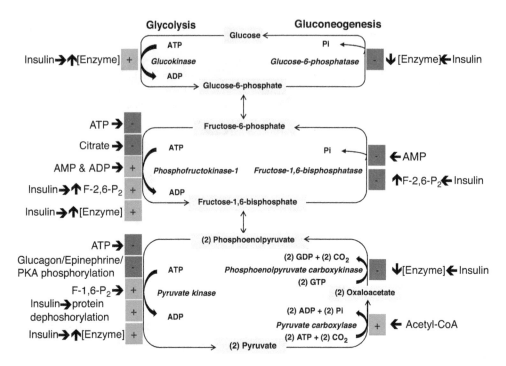

Figure 10.12: **Figure 10.12: Allosteric, Transcriptional, and Covalent Regulation of Glycolysis and Gluconeogenesis.** [Enzyme] denotes an increase or decrease in transcription of that enzyme.

presence of insulin also decreases the transcription of glucose-6 phosphatase[7] and PEPCK[5], thereby decreasing the presence of gluconeogenesis enzymes.

The last regulation of gluconeogenesis/glycolysis is through covalent modification (phosphorylation) of pyruvate kinase. In the presence of insulin, PP1, will dephosphorylate pyruvate kinase, driving glycolysis. In presence of glucagon, PKA will phosphorylate pyruvate kinase, blocking its activity, and thereby blocking glycolysis, allowing gluconeogenesis to proceed. A summary of the regulation between glycolysis and gluconeogenesis can be seen in Figure 10.12.

Ketogenesis

In a fasted state, fatty acids are the primary substrate for energy and during a prolonged fast (> 24 hours), beta oxidation of fatty acids is crucial to spare blood glucose. Remember that the product of beta oxidation is acetyl CoA, which enters the TCA cycle. Acetyl CoA is also the building block of ketones. The rate of beta oxidation is proportional to the rate of ketone production. That means that individuals eating a high carbohydrate diet would generally have low ketone production. However, for those individuals that are in a prolonged fast, ketone levels will increase. In addition, individuals on low (very low) carbohydrate diets would also have elevated ketone levels, as well as individuals who are undertaking prolonged exercise without replenishing their carbohydrates (ex. during a marathon). Finally, individuals with uncontrolled diabetes, where there is pancreatic beta cell failure, would have elevated ketone levels alongside increased blood glucose levels, called diabetic ketoacidosis.

There are three forms of ketones. Both D-3-hydroxybutyrate and acetoacetate are made in the mitochondria of liver cells (hepatocytes). A third form, acetone, is formed in the blood by spontaneous decarboxylation of acetoacetate (Figure 10.13). All three forms can be taken up by cells that have mitochondria, and be broken back down into acetyl CoA, which can then feed into the TCA cycle for oxidation phosphorylation.

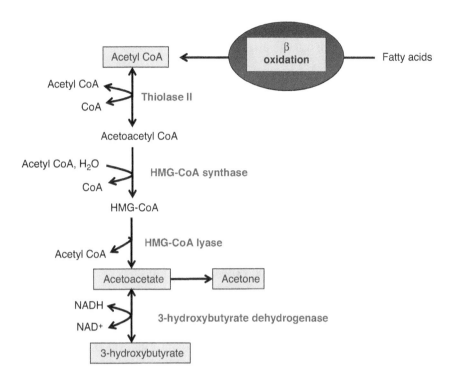

Figure 10.13: **Ketogenesis – the Process**. The first 2 steps (formation of HMG CoA from acetyl CoA) are the same enzymes used in cholesterol synthesis. The key difference is that in cholesterol synthesis, this process takes place in the cytosol and in ketogenesis, it takes place in the mitochondria. This compartmentalizes the two pathways and prevents competition for acetyl CoA. The final product in the liver is 3-hydroxybutyrate, a ketone.

Why make these ketones anyway? It is thought that during famine, the body developed this method to produce ketones to "replace" the need for glucose use by cells with mitochondria. For example, in brain cells, which need a lot of glucose, approximately 60% of the energy can be derived from ketones during fasting. Think about this—when glucose is low and glycogen stores are low, only gluconeogenesis is being used to produce glucose to maintain blood glucose levels. Fats are then being used for energy, and in this case, with the production of the acetyl CoA, ketones can be produced. Any cell with mitochondria can use ketones to produce ATP, and as ketone use goes up, the need for glucose goes down from ~5 grams/hour to ~1 gram/hour. This is a significant savings to the body. In addition, a decreased reliance on glucose, spares muscle degradation for amino acid precursors for gluconeogenesis.

Ketones are water soluble and are produced in the liver—however the liver does not have the enzymes to oxidize ketones thereby preventing a futile cycle of production and oxidation. The liver is 100% reliant on fatty acid oxidation for the production of ketones, and therefore is reliant on getting these fatty acids from lipolysis in the adipose tissue. After 24 hours of starvation, ketogenesis ramps up, as fatty acids are high (due to increased lipolysis in the adipose tissue). As the liver is oxidizing fatty acids through beta oxidation, it is also producing large amounts of acetyl CoA, and the surplus will be shuttled to ketogenesis. Ketogenesis in fact, also occurs in mitochondria where the acetyl CoA is being consumed, which is pretty efficient in that the acetyl CoA not used, can be directly shuttled over to ketogenesis.

How is this done? First, two acetyl CoA molecules are converted to acetoacetyl CoA using the enzyme thiolase II (or acetoacetyl-CoA thiolase) (Figure 10.13). A third acetyl CoA then is added, producing 3-hydroxyl-3-methylglutaryl CoA (HMG-CoA), by the enzyme HMG-CoA reductase. These first two steps are actually the exact same as the steps for the production of cholesterol. The main difference is that cholesterol synthesis takes place in the cytoplasm, whereas ketogenesis is taking place in the mitochondria. This compartmentalization of the two processes means that there is no real competition for the substrate. As we continue in the process of ketogenesis, HMG-CoA is split to form acetoacetate and an acetyl CoA, by HMG-CoA lyase. The acetoacetate can be converted, spontaneously into acetone and a CO_2 in the blood, or with the help of the 3-hydroxybutyrate dehydrogenase enzyme and one NADH, it can be energetically converted to 3-hydroxybutyrate (Figure 10.13).

> ### "Sweet"-smelling breath of carbohydrate starvation
>
> Acetone produced during this process is highly volatile, and sweet smelling. Exhalation of acetone is responsible for the unique smell on the breath of a person with high ketones. So, if you decide to go on a low carb diet, use some (sugar-free) breath mints!

Like many of the other metabolic processes that we have talked about, ketogenesis is also regulated. Remember that when insulin is present, it leads to dephosphorylation of lipolysis enzymes, thereby decreasing lipolysis and the supply of fatty acids to the liver. On the other hand, glucagon works to allow fatty acid entry into the mitochondria by activation of AMPK and subsequent phosphorylation of acetyl CoA carboxylase (ACC2) thereby inhibiting it, allowing for the removal of malonyl CoA (which is actively blocking CPT1) by an active malonyl CoA decarboxylase (MCD).

Oxidation of Ketone Bodies

Once made in the liver, ketones are released into the blood as fuel sources for the brain, muscle, and other energy needy tissues. During fasting, the concentration of ketones becomes higher in blood than in the tissues, allowing the tissues to take up the ketones along a concentration gradient. Once taken up into the tissues, ketones (D-3-hydroxybutyrate, most commonly referred to as beta-hydroxybutyrate) are broken down to acetoacetate, and then acetoacetyl CoA, which can further be metabolized to two acetyl CoA molecules (Figure 10.14). Note that this process does require the use of NAD^+. The two acetyl CoA molecules can then enter the TCA cycle and be oxidized, providing sources of ATP and NADH needed by energy starved tissues.

Ketogenesis versus ketoacidosis

Ketogenesis is the process of making ketones and it is normal; we all do it at some level when in between meals, or after having a lower carbohydrate meal. However, ketoacidosis is a pathological process that refers to the acidification of blood due to such high levels of ketones in circulation. Ketoacidosis can occur in an uncontrolled diabetic state. This is especially true with Type 1 diabetics who are unable to produce insulin, and therefore cannot use glucose like a non-diabetic. Type 2 diabetics who are uncontrolled (i.e. not secreting enough insulin to control the levels of glucose) can also end up in ketoacidosis.

To look at this more in detail, a state of hypoinsulinemia will lead to hyperglycemia. There is significant loss of water and electrolytes during kidney filtration due to an overall change in the osmolality of the blood. This condition is called glycosuria, and characterized by high urine output, and high urine glucose, leading to dehydration. Increased dehydration leads to excessive thirst, and a condition known as hypovolemia, which is essentially reduced blood volume, and can also increase circulating lactate, possibly due

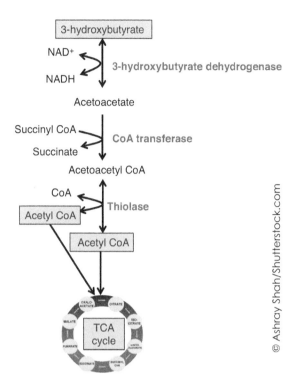

Figure 10.14: **Oxidation of Ketone Bodies.** D-3-hydroxybutyrate is oxidized to acetoacetate, which is then converted into acetoacetate and then acetoacetyl CoA, finally producing two acetyl CoAs that can enter the TCA cycle.

to hypoperfusion of tissues. The reduced blood volume and increased lactate signals the body to take counter-regulatory measures—namely increasing glucagon, cortisol, growth hormone, and epinephrine. Cortisol and epinephrine have been discussed before—but in fact, all of these are going to tip the balance in tissues from generating energy from fats and carbohydrates, to mobilizing fats (from adipose tissue) and degrading proteins (from muscle), and producing ketones (in the liver) (Figure 10.15). Together these will increase acidosis, which unfortunately, feeds right back into the counter regulatory measures—increasing glucagon, cortisol, growth hormone, and epinephrine. And so, the cycle continues.

Ketogenic diet

The ketogenic diet emerged in modern history in the 1920s for the treatment of epilepsy by physicians[8]. However, the prescription of a ketogenic diet fell out of vogue for treatment of epilepsy with the introduction of prescription medications in 1938[8]. But in 1972, Dr. Robert Atkins, a cardiologist, released his book, "Dr. Atkins' Diet Revolution" for losing weight[9]. Since the popularization of the Atkins' diet, many other

You didn't say...

While osmolarity and osmolality both refer to units of measurement, os<u>molar</u>ity is the osmoles (in 6.02 x 10^{23} particles per osmole) of something (in this case glucose) per liter of solution, while os<u>molal</u>ity is the number of osmoles in a kilogram of solute. Osmolality is used to describe the <u>concentration of particles</u> in a solution (mmol/kg), while osmolarity is used to describe the <u>number of particles</u> in the solution (mmol/L). The normal osmolarity of plasma and other body fluids is ~300 mmol/L, while normal plasma osmolality is ~295 mmol/kg. These are very similar, which makes sense because plasma is usually very dilute, like water, and water's density is 1 kg/L. So, in human physiology, these terms are sometimes interchanged.

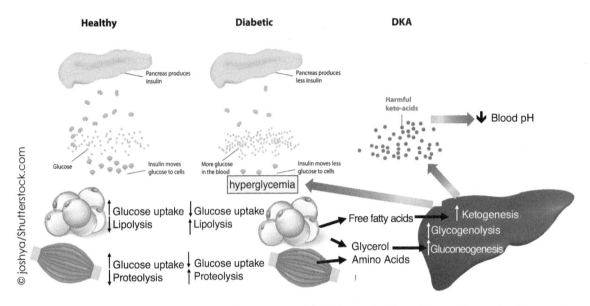

Figure 10.15: **Insufficient Insulin Productions, as seen in Diabetes leads to Hyperglycemia.** Elevated glucose in the blood leads to excretion of glucose in urine (glucosuria), as well as water and electrolytes, which together lead to a decreased blood volume (hypovolemia). A decreased blood volume results in an endocrine response of stress hormones and decreased tissue perfusion, leading to increased lactate production. Lipolysis in adipose tissue and proteolysis in muscle provide gluconeogenic precursors. High levels of beta oxidation in the liver results in an increase in ketone formation. Both increased lactate and ketones in the blood can lead to acidification of the blood (acidosis), known as diabetic ketoacidosis (DKA).

low-carbohydrate diets have been introduced in hopes of rapid and substantial weight-loss. Only the first restrictive phase of the Atkins' diet mirrors the ketogenic diet, as a traditional ketogenic diet is very low in carbohydrates[9]. So, from a health and weight loss perspective, what is the rationale behind a ketogenic diet? We all know someone who has tried one (or maybe you have tried one yourself) and sees very accelerated weight loss, especially initially. However, energy balance is still key for long term weight management. In many controlled feeding studies, energy balance, rather than macronutrient composition is what determines whether the individual gains or loses weight[10].

Take for example two people each with a deficit of 500 kcals in their diet. One is on a ketogenic diet, and one is just on a lower calorie diet. Who will lose more weight? Who will feel better about "dieting"? There is evidence to suggest that higher protein, lower carbohydrate diets suppress hunger, and that ketones directly can also suppress hunger. In addition, research has shown less attrition for those on a ketogenic diet versus a low-fat diet. However, when these studies have been done in a very controlled setting, those on a low-fat diet lose more body fat, but those on a low-carbohydrate diet lose more weight[11]. But in both diets, there was a significant loss of body weight and body fat than prior to the intervention. Is one diet better than the other?

> ### Measurement of Ketones
>
> Many websites promoting a ketogenic diet, recommend concentration of blood ketones somewhere in the range of 0.5 – 3 mM. But always check with your doctor first before starting a new diet! How would you measure your blood ketone levels?
>
> - Over the counter urine tests measure acetoacetate, but could underestimate overall ketone levels, since acetoacetate is commonly reduced to beta-hydroxybutyrate during times of increased ketogenesis.
> - Over the counter finger prick kits that measure beta-hydroxybutyrate.

Proteolysis in prolonged fasting and starvation

What about proteins? In a post-meal phase, protein degradation is part of the normal process. However, large-scale protein degradation can and will occur during prolonged fasting. Between 24–48 hours of fasting, blood cortisol levels rise, stimulating proteolysis of muscle. Remember that the carbon skeletons of amino acids can be shuttled into gluconeogenesis, the TCA cycle, and ketogenesis (see **Figure 5.2**). As starvation progresses beyond ~48 hours, proteolysis decreases and ketone production increases—this is a means to preserve body protein as it may be needed later as an energy source.

In addition, the urea cycle is needed when protein degradation is taking place, as the build-up of nitrogen can be toxic—but the urea cycle takes care of these, helping to neutralize, and move the nitrogen out and into urea. As we talked about in chapter 5, the body then has two ways to deal with ammonium and to clear it out of the body—the urea cycle, and production of glutamine from glutamate using the enzyme glutamate synthetase. As seen in Figure 5.6, there are five key enzymes that are a part of the urea cycle. As nitrogen levels in the body increase, the genes of these enzymes are transcriptionally upregulated, producing more enzymes to meet urea cycle demand. In addition, the first enzyme in the cycle, carbamoyl phosphate synthetase 1 (CPS1) is also regulated allosterically. If the cycle begins to slow, arginine allosterically activates the enzyme N-acetyl glutamate synthase, which converts an acetyl CoA and a glutamate amino acid into N-acetyl glutamate (NAG). It is NAG then, that allosterically activates CPS1, thereby increasing its activity and consequently the rate of urea formation in the urea cycle.

Summary

To summarize, during fasting (and eventually starvation), the level of blood glucose will decrease, and in fact, by about 12 hours past the last meal, blood glucose levels will be at their minimum. The body at this point is doing everything it can to defend blood glucose levels, because if they drop too far, the brain will not be able to carry out its functions, and the organism will die. However, first, using glycogen stores via glycogenolysis, and then creating new glucose via gluconeogenesis, blood glucose levels can be kept at the minimum level needed to maintain life (Figure 10.16). However, there is a limit to this, and it has to do with how "full" the stores of proteins, triglycerides, and lactate are available to make the pyruvate, oxaloacetate, and glycerol as substrates for gluconeogenesis. Without these, gluconeogenesis will slow down and eventually stop, and the organism will no longer be able to maintain blood glucose levels, with death ensuing.

To spare blood glucose, fatty acid metabolism dominates. In response to glucagon and catecholamines, lipolysis in adipose tissue is active, providing free fatty acids for beta oxidation and ATP production. The presence of these hormones also causes glycolysis to slow, which will allow gluconeogenesis to proceed as needed. As the fasting continues, high rates of beta oxidation lead to ketogenesis, which also spares blood glucose by providing an alternative substrate for energy. In addition, cortisol levels rise leading to muscle proteolysis and the freeing of amino acids for either anaplerosis (replenishing of TCA cycle intermediates), carbon skeletons for gluconeogenesis, or acetyl CoA for ketogenesis. In fact, you can think of the TCA cycle as central to many if not all the energy metabolism processes in the body. Think about it—glycolysis, beta-oxidation, ketogenesis, and proteolysis all feed into the TCA cycle.

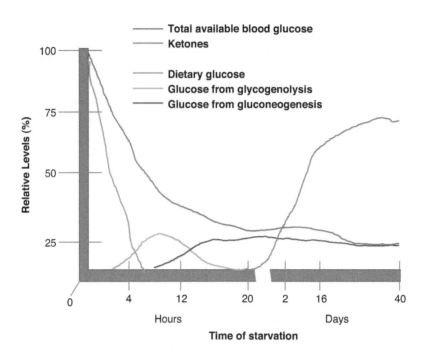

Figure 10.16: Glucose Sources During a Fed, Fasted, Prolonged fast, and Starvation. As we move from the fed to fasted state, blood glucose levels drop (red line) and dietary glucose sources move to zero (orange line). Liver glycogenolysis then increases to maintain blood glucose (green line). As we enter a prolonged fast and into starvation, glycogen stores are depleted (green line), gluconeogenesis increases and is essential to maintain blood glucose (purple line), and ketones become an important energy source to spare blood glucose (blue line).

Points to Ponder

➤ How long could a 500 lb. male survive without food compared to a 150 lb. male? Would the process of starvation be the same for each man?
➤ Do you think a ketogenic diet is a healthy way to lose weight? Are there risks involved?
➤ Would adhering to a ketogenic diet affect exercise performance for endurance athletes? How about anaerobic athletes like sprinters and weight lifters?
➤ What do you think the trigger is for cortisol release in a fasted state?

References

1. Vance ML, Thorner MO. Fasting alters pulsatile and rhythmic cortisol release in normal man. *J Clin Endocrinol Metab.* 1989;68(6):1013–1018.
2. Pettersson J, Hindorf U, Persson P, et al. Muscular exercise can cause highly pathological liver function tests in healthy men. *Br J Clin Pharmacol.* 2008;65(2):253–259.
3. Assimacopoulos-Jeannet F, Jeanrenaud B. Insulin activates 6-phosphofructo-2-kinase and pyruvate kinase in the liver. Indirect evidence for an action via a phosphatase. *J Biol Chem.* 1990;265(13):7202–7206.
4. Lemaigre FP, Rousseau GG. Transcriptional control of genes that regulate glycolysis and gluconeogenesis in adult liver. *Biochem J.* 1994;303 (Pt 1):1–14.
5. Meisler MH, Howard G. Effects of insulin on gene transcription. *Annu Rev Physiol.* 1989;51:701–714.
6. Pilkis SJ, Granner DK. Molecular physiology of the regulation of hepatic gluconeogenesis and glycolysis. *Annu Rev Physiol.* 1992;54:885–909.

7. Nordlie RC, Foster JD, Lange AJ. Regulation of glucose production by the liver. *Annu Rev Nutr.* 1999;19:379–406.

8. Wheless JW. History of the ketogenic diet. *Epilepsia.* 2008;49 Suppl 8:3–5.

9. Booth F. Effects of endurance exercise on cytochrome C turnover in skeletal muscle. *Ann N Y Acad Sci.* 1977;301:431–439.

10. Sacks FM, Bray GA, Carey VJ, et al. Comparison of weight-loss diets with different compositions of fat, protein, and carbohydrates. *N Engl J Med.* 2009;360(9):859–873.

11. Hall KD, Bemis T, Brychta R, et al. Calorie for Calorie, Dietary Fat Restriction Results in More Body Fat Loss than Carbohydrate Restriction in People with Obesity. *Cell Metab.* 2015;22(3):427–436.

CHAPTER 11

Metabolic Flexibility

Metabolic Flexibility

What does the term metabolic flexibility mean? Basically, we've been talking about metabolic flexibility all along because this term refers to our body's ability to shift back and forth and modulate fuel oxidation based on fuel availability. In the short term, when we are full, or in the fed state, we will shift to glucose oxidation because it is the fuel that is most available. Conversely, when we are fasted, fatty acid oxidation predominates. In the long term, there is an adaptation of fuel oxidation based on daily, long term, habitual food (macronutrient) intake. For example, if someone is on a high fat diet for the long term and if metabolic flexibility is maintained, then fatty acid oxidation will predominate in this person. However, (and unfortunately) in some cases, as we'll see later, individuals become "metabolically inflexible" and can't modulate their metabolism based on intake.

RQ and RER

How do we determine which macronutrient is being metabolized? We do this by measuring consumption of O_2 as the volume per minute of O_2 (called VO_2), and the production of CO_2, measured again in volume per minute and referred to as VCO_2. Why CO_2 and O_2? Because during glucose oxidation we use 6 O_2 molecules and produce 6 CO_2 molecules, but during oxidation of the fatty acid palmitic acid (as an example), these numbers are much different, with 23 O_2 molecules used and 16 CO_2 molecules produced. During normal physiology, oxygen is inhaled; it then circulates in the blood and is taken up by metabolically active cells and used by the electron transport chain. Carbon dioxide on the other hand is produced directly through metabolism in the PDH reaction and the TCA cycle, it then circulates in blood until it is exhaled. The measure of metabolic flexibility is the ratio between the CO_2 exhaled and the O_2 consumed, which is referred to as the respiratory quotient (RQ)–which is the correct term when measurements are made at the cellular or organ level via arterial and venous catheterizations, or the respiratory exchange ratio (RER), which is the correct term when measurements are made using exhaled and inhaled breaths (refer back to chapter 1).

Based on the measurements that are made (Figure 11.1), one can determine if the person is predominately utilizing carbs (1.0 RQ), or fats (0.7 RQ). Most people do not show these exact values, but end up somewhere is the middle, between 0.83–0.85 indicating that they are using about 50% carbohydrates and a 50% fat, and of course these values vary during the day depending on whether someone is fed or fasted. After a prolonged fast, when fat oxidation predominates, the measured RER or RQ level will decrease to around 0.7. On the other hand, with a 100% carbohydrate meal, the RQ/RER will rise to be closer to 1.0. Finally, when someone is at

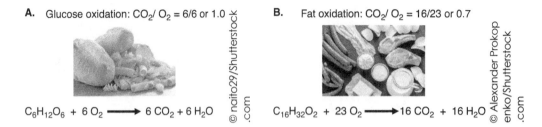

A. Glucose oxidation: $CO_2/O_2 = 6/6$ or 1.0

$$C_6H_{12}O_6 + 6\,O_2 \longrightarrow 6\,CO_2 + 6\,H_2O$$

© naito29/Shutterstock.com

B. Fat oxidation: $CO_2/O_2 = 16/23$ or 0.7

$$C_{16}H_{32}O_2 + 23\,O_2 \longrightarrow 16\,CO_2 + 16\,H_2O$$

© Alexander Prokopenko/Shutterstock.com

Figure 11.1: **Stoichiometry for Glucose and Fatty Acid Oxidation.** (**A**) It takes 6 O_2 to catabolize glucose, producing 6 CO_2 molecules. So when oxidizing only carbohydrates, the RER/RQ ratio would be 1.0. (**B**) It takes 23 O_2 molecules to catabolize a 16 carbon fatty acid, producing 16 CO_2 molecules. So when oxidizing only fats, the RER/RQ ratio would be 0.7.

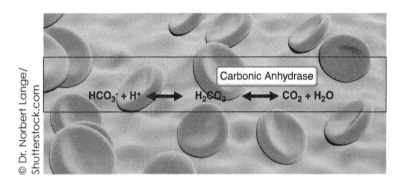

© Dr. Norbert Lange/Shutterstock.com

Carbonic Anhydrase

$$HCO_3^- + H^+ \longleftrightarrow H_2CO_3 \longleftrightarrow CO_2 + H_2O$$

Figure 11.2: **The Bicarbonate System.** When lactate is produced, the process releases a H^+ ion into the blood. High amounts of lactate can acidify the blood, therefore the presence of the bicarbonate system buffers the lowering pH. Bicarbonate combines with the H^+, making carbonic acid. Carbonic acid is then acted upon by carbonic anhydrase, producing CO_2 and H_2O. This process traps the H^+ ions as harmless water. However, this process also produces CO_2 that needs to be exhaled at the lungs.

their "VO$_2$ max" during exercise, and there is a lot of lactate in circulation, the RQ/RER can rise to around 1.1, which is indicative that someone has reached their maximum output. The reason is that in solution lactate can release a proton (H^+), which can lower blood pH. The body buffers the protons with the bicarbonate system. The proton combines with bicarbonate to produce carbonic acid. Carbonic acid then disassociates via carbonic anhydrase to form CO_2 and H_2O, thereby trapping the proton as water and the body then exhales the CO_2 (Figure 11.2). You can see then, that if the bicarbonate system is highly active, the amount of CO_2 exhaled, can increase thereby increasing the RQ/RER above 1.0.

An RQ/RER above a 1.0 can also occur in a non-exercise state when *de novo* fatty acid synthesis is occurring. Let's look at the process a little more closely. As you remember from chapter 7 (see **Figure 7.12**), two key enzymes acetyl CoA carboxylase (ACC1) and fatty acid synthetase (FAS) are needed. But FAS is actually seven different enzymes rolled into one, along with a protein carrier, acyl carrier protein (ACP), which shuttles the growing fatty acid to the active sites of the ACP-dependent enzymes in FAS. Figure 11.3 shows the FAS enzyme complex and where the different enzymes are located.

When the 2-carbon acetyl CoA (formed into acetyl-ACP via acetyl transcylase) and the 3-carbon malonyl CoA (formed into malonyl-ACP via malonyl transcylase), known collectively as MAT, are condensed together via β-keto acyl synthase (KS), a CO_2 is released in the process, forming a 4-carbon molecule. This molecule goes through several other changes via enzymes 4–6 (β-keto acyl reductase (KR), (β-hydroxy acyl dehydratase (DH), Enoyl reductase (ER)) listed in Figure 11.3, preparing the 4-carbon molecule to accept another malonyl CoA and proceed through the enzymatic steps 2–6 another time. Again, when step 3 is reached β-keto acyl synthase (KS) condenses the

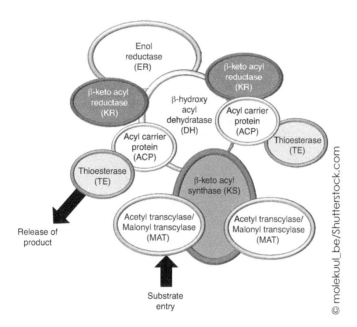

© molekuul_be/Shutterstock.com

Figure 11.3: **Fatty Acid Synthetase.** Cartoon version of Fatty acid synthetase (FAS). This enzyme is made up of 7 separate enzymes, as well as an acyl carrier protein (ACP), that shuttles the developing fatty acid to the active site of ACP-dependent enzymes. The enzymes that make up FAS are Acetyl transferase (AT), Malonyl transferase (MT), β-keto acyl synthase (KS), β-keto acyl reductase (KR), β-hydroxy acyl dehydratase (DH), Enoyl reductase (ER), and Thioesterase (TE). ER, DH, and KS are homodimers, although in the cartoon they appear as only one enzyme.

growing chain with the malonyl-ACP and releases another CO_2. So, to form the 16:0 fatty acid, palmitate, 7 CO_2 molecules are produced in the process. You can see why *de novo* fatty acid synthesis could raise the RQ/RER above 1.0 as well. You might have noticed that there was no mention of the last enzyme, thioesterase. Thioesterase's (TE) job is to release the finished fatty acid from FAS.

Glucose-Fatty Acid Cycle

Unless you know Jack Sprat and his wife, (from the English nursery rhyme), most people do not eat all fat, or all carbohydrates, but rather have a mixed meal. Thus, as shown on Figure 11.4A/B, the RER or RQ (depending on how the measurement is being done) will vary during the day in response to the rise and fall in blood glucose levels. This rise and fall in RER/RQ *is metabolic flexibility*; it is the ability to vary substrate oxidation depending on fuel availability. After a meal, blood glucose will rise and metabolism switches to the oxidation of glucose. In between meals, or in a fasted state, blood glucose is conserved and metabolism switches to the oxidation of fatty acids. However, if an individual does not show this rise and fall, or has a muted response to changes in fuel availability, then they are considered *metabolically inflexible.*

> Fun Fact
>
> Phillip Randle was born in the same English county as William Shakespeare. *To be or not to be…*in metabolic flexibility. *That is the question!*

The glucose-fatty acid cycle was first proposed by Randle and colleagues in 1963[1], and became known as the Randle Cycle. In this publication, Randle proposed that glucose and fatty acids *compete* for oxidation, so that when there are high levels of glucagon present, catabolic pathways would dominate. Conversely, when there are high levels of insulin present, then anabolic pathways would dominate. Remember that at the time, sophisticated methods for measuring RER or RQ were not available, so much of what Randle proposed was a hypothesis. However, as of today, more than 50 years in the future, the Randle

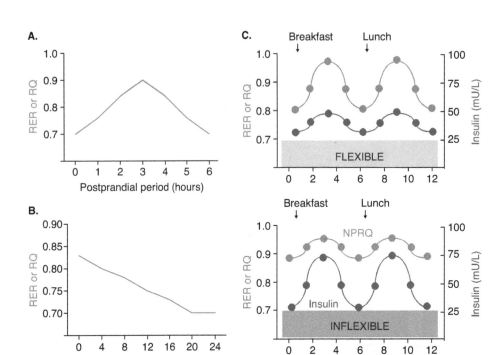

Figure 11.4: **Metabolic Flexibility.** (A) In a metabolically flexible person during the postprandial period (fed state), blood glucose rises and therefore metabolism switches to glucose oxidation raising the RER/RQ post meal. (B) In a metabolically flexible person in a fasted state, blood glucose is conserved and metabolism switches to fatty acid oxidation lowering the RQ/RER. A and B were adapted from Kelley and colleagues (1999), referenced in text. (C) Comparison of Non-protein respiratory quotient (NPRQ, green line) and insulin flux (blue line) for both a metabolically flexible and a metabolically inflexible individual over a 12 hour period with meals and post-prandial periods (derived from Bergouignan and colleagues, (2013), referenced in text.

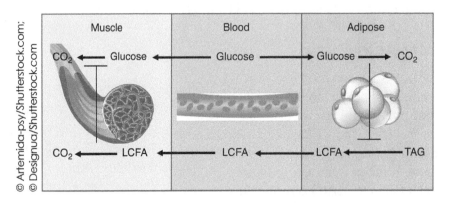

Figure 11.5: **The Glucose- Fatty Acid Cycle.** When blood glucose is high (top row), glucose oxidation is favored in muscle and adipose tissue. High glucose levels inhibit lipolysis (TAG → LCFA) in adipose tissue. When blood glucose is low, levels of long chain fatty acids (LCFAs) rise in the blood (bottom row) due to lipolysis from triglycerides (TAG) in adipose tissue. These LCFAs are taken up in muscle for oxidation and this high fatty acid flux into the cell, inhibits glucose oxidation.

cycle still prevails as the model for metabolic flexibility. You can see this more clearly in a diagram derived from a paper by Hue and colleagues,[2] which was published in 2009 (Figure 11.5). During a fed-state, blood glucose levels are high and favor glucose metabolism. The favoring of glucose metabolism in adipose tissue then blocks lipolysis, decreasing circulating fatty acids. Conversely, during a fasted state where blood glucose levels are low, lipolysis now can proceed and the presence of long chain fatty acids

(LCFAs) in circulation rises. These fatty acids are taken-up by muscle, where fatty acid oxidation dominates, thereby blocking glucose oxidation. The cycle really functions in the short-term…in other words, using allosteric and covalent changes that lead to flexibility. On the other hand, longer-term changes in diet are manipulated by the body using transcriptional mechanisms, with changes in the total amounts of proteins for certain key pathways. We still are learning though how short- and long-term changes occur, and identifying "all the moving parts" of these metabolic flexibility pathways.

Regulation of the Glucose-Fatty Acid Cycle

What are the important control points? We can name five key enzymes that provide points of regulation: pyruvate dehydrogenase (PDH), phosphofructokinase 1 (PFK1), hexokinase (HK)/ Glucokinase (GK), acetyl CoA carboxylase (ACC), and malonyl CoA decarboxylase (MCD). Let's talk about each of these and review the pathways they are involved in, focusing on how each of these enzymes are a pivotal point in metabolism.

Pyruvate Dehydrogenase

PDH functions as the bridge between glycolysis and the TCA cycle, taking pyruvate and making acetyl CoA inside the mitochondria. As you remember, levels of acetyl CoA determine the activity of the TCA cycle. Thus, PDH plays an important regulatory step in glucose metabolism, and therefore is a target of regulation (Figure 11.6). In fact, changes to PDH are made allosterically and by covalently modulating the enzyme through phosphorylation. PDH can be phosphorylated by PDH kinase (PDK), resulting in *inactivation* of the enzyme, whereas PDH phosphatase (PDP) can de-phosphorylate PDH, resulting in *activation* of PDH. Within the PDH enzyme, there are three possible places

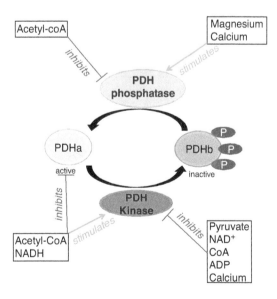

Figure 11.6: **Regulation of Pyruvate Dehydrogenase (PDH).** PDH is allosterically inhibited by acetyl CoA and NADH. In addition, PDH can be phosphorylated (P) by pyruvate dehydrogenase kinase (PDK), thereby inhibiting PDH (PDHb). PDK is allosterically activated by acetyl CoA and NADH. PDK is allosterically inhibited by pyruvate, NAD+, CoA, ADP, and calcium. PDH can be dephosphorylated by pyruvate dehydrogenase phosphatase (PDP), activating PDH (PDHa). PDP is allosterically inhibited by acetyl CoA and allosterically activated by magnesium and calcium.

that can be phosphorylated, with higher phosphorylation correlating with less activity. In addition, the enzymes that covalently modify PDH themselves can be turned on and off allosterically.

PDK, for example, is activated by elevations in acetyl CoA and by elevations in NADH—and as you hopefully recall, these also both allosterically inhibit PDH (Figure 11.6). On the other hand, high levels of pyruvate, NAD^+, ADP, or calcium can inhibit PDK. This makes sense, right? When we have high substrate or energy demand, we want PDH to be activate, and therefore we want PDK *not* to phosphorylate PDH. What about PDP? Based on the scenario above, can you guess? You should have said that acetyl CoA would inhibit PDP, while magnesium and calcium (perhaps signaling exercise, especially in muscle where calcium would be released), would stimulate PDP and result in a dephosphorylation and an active PDH enzyme (Figure 11.6).

Phosphofructokinase

As you may remember from our discussions of glycolysis, PFK1 is the major regulator of rate of glycolysis. PFK1 is regulated allosterically, with AMP, ADP, and fructose 2,6-bisphosphate (F2,6BP) allosterically activating PFK1. This make sense, right? When AMP/ADP levels are rising, this signifies an energy demand and the rate of glycolysis needs to increase. You may not remember where F2,6BP comes from. F2,6BP is the product of PFK2, which is allosterically activated by AMP—again signifying an energy demand. PFK2 is crucial in the liver, due to its pivotal role in regulating glycolysis versus gluconeogenesis. So, it would make sense then that products signifying adequate rates of glycolysis would allosterically inhibit PFK1 and that is the case. Both ATP and citrate feedback on PFK1, decreasing its activity, and thereby decreasing the rate of glycolysis (see **Figure 10.12**).

Hexokinase/Glucokinase

Hexokinase (HK), the isoform found in muscle, is the enzyme that converts glucose coming into the cell to glucose-6-phosphate (G6P). Glucokinase (GK), the isoform found in the liver and pancreas, does this same job. We have talked previously about how both hexokinase and glucokinase are regulated. To refresh, the product of HK, G6P allosterically inhibits HK, slowing down the reaction. For GK in the liver, it is regulated by being sequestered by GK regulatory protein (GKRP) that keeps it in the nucleus when glucose levels are low. As glucose and insulin levels rise, GKRP releases GK, which can migrate to the cytoplasm and phosphorylate glucose to G6P (See **Figure 7.5**).

Acetyl CoA Carboxylase and Malonyl CoA Decarboxylase

Acetyl CoA carboxylase (ACC) has two main isoforms: ACC1 and ACC2. Both do the same job of converting acetyl CoA to malonyl CoA. Malonyl CoA has two main functions. The first is as the building block for fatty acid synthesis (see RQ/RER section about *de novo* fatty acid synthesis). The second is that malonyl CoA blocks the mitochondrial fatty acid transporter—carnitine palmitoyl transferase (CPT1), also known as carnitine acyl transferase (CAT1). When CPT1 is blocked, fatty acids cannot enter the mitochondria and glucose oxidation is predominate. Due to differential expression of the two isoforms, ACC1 is found in lipogenic tissues and is for fatty acid synthesis, where ACC2 is found in muscle and other tissues where regulation of fatty acid oxidation is important. We'll be talking about ACC2 here in terms of how malonyl CoA is a crucial part of regulating the glucose-fatty acid cycle.

So, how is ACC2 regulated? ACC2 is regulated both allosterically and covalently. In fact, ACC2 is one of those enzymes that is active in the dephosphorylated state. Consequently, when insulin is present, it activates protein phosphatases that dephosphorylate ACC2 making it active. This makes sense, right? When insulin is present, we are in a fed state and we want glucose oxidation to

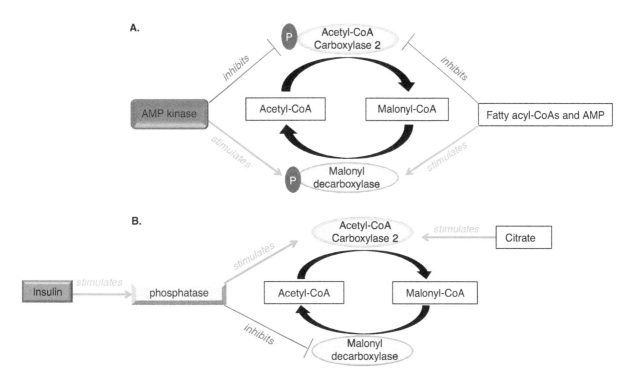

Figure 11.7: **Regulation of Acetyl CoA Carboxylase (ACC) and Malonyl CoA Decarboxylase (MCD).**
A. AMP kinase (AMPK), active in times of energy demand, phosphorylates acetyl CoA carboxylase 2
(ACC2), inhibiting it, and phosphorylates malony CoA decarboxylase (MCD), activating it, allowing for
the conversion of malonyl CoA to acetyl CoA, reducing the block of carnitine palmitoyl transferase (CPT1)
by malonyl CoA. Fatty acids also allosterically inhibit ACC and activate MCD. **B.** The presence of insulin
activates protein phosphatases that dephosphorylate ACC, activating it, and dephosphorylates MCD, inhibiting
it, allowing for the conversion of acetyl CoA to malonyl CoA, which blocks CPT1, thereby fatty acid entrance
into the mitochondria. ACC is also allosterically activated by citrate and inhibited by palmitoyl CoA and AMP.

proceed, so we want ACC2 producing malonyl CoA to block CPT1 and consequently fatty acid oxidation. ACC2 is also allosterically activated by citrate—blocking fatty acid entry to the mitochondria by producing malonyl CoA so that glucose oxidation can proceed. Remember, citrate is also an
allosteric activator of PFK1, which drives glucose oxidation. ACC2 is inhibited by phosphorylation,
specifically by AMPK (look back at **Figure 10.8** for a reminder on how this works) and allosterically inhibited by fatty acids and AMP. This makes sense that during energy demands, when fatty
acids are present, we would want to get them into the mitochondria for oxidation, as well as increase
the amount of acetyl CoA for ATP production.

Malonyl-CoA decarboxylase (MCD) is the enzyme that works opposite ACC2 and is therefore
regulated in the opposite way (Figure 11.7). MCD converts malonyl CoA to acetyl CoA, thereby
removing the block on CPT1, allowing for fatty acids to enter the mitochondria and fatty acid oxidation to proceed. Since it works opposite ACC2, it is active when phosphorylated and inactive when
dephosphorylated. At the same time protein phosphatases are dephosphorylating ACC2, activating
it, they are also dephosphorylating MCD, inhibiting the enzymatic activity[3]. Likewise, when AMPK
is phosphorylating ACC2, inhibiting its activity, AMPK is also phosphorylating MCD making it
active[3]. It makes sense that under energy demand (when AMPK is active), MCD would be active
converting malonyl CoA to acetyl CoA, making it available for ATP production. Fatty acids also
allosterically activate MCD, allowing for a reduction in malonyl CoA and opening of CPT1 for fatty
acid transport (Figure 11.7).

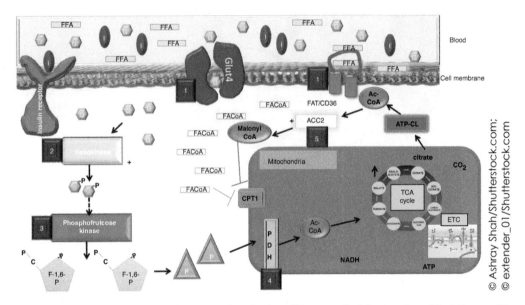

Figure 11.8: Summary of Regulatory Factors that Drive Glucose Oxidation in a Fed State. The presence of insulin (I) leads to GLUT4 and FAT/CD36 translocation (Regulatory step #1) and glucose (G) and fatty acid (FACoA) entry. Hexokinase (Regulatory step #2) converts G to glucose-6-phosphate (G6P), which proceeds through glycolysis or is stored as glycogen. Allosteric inhibitors of phosphofructokinase 1 (PFK1) are not present and F 2,6 BP can also allosterically activate PFK1 (Regulatory step #3), allowing the production of fructose 1,6 bisphosphate (F-1,6BP) and eventually pyruvate (P). Pyruvate enters the mitochondria. Pyruvate dehydrogenase (PDH) (Regulatory step #4) is not inhibited by pyruvate dehydrogenase kinase (PDK), thereby allowing the production of acetyl CoA (Ac-CoA). As acetyl CoA builds, some is shuttled out of the mitochondria as citrate via the citrate shuttle. Citrate is converted back to acetyl CoA in the cytoplasm by ATP-citrate lyase (ATP-CL). The presence of insulin also activates protein phosphatases that dephosphorylate acetyl CoA carboxylase (ACC2) and malonyl CoA decarboxylase (MCD), making ACC2 active (Regulatory step #5), which converts acetyl CoA to malonyl CoA. Malonyl CoA then blocks carnitine palmitoyl transporter 1 (CPT1), which blocks fatty acid entry into the mitochondria and subsequent fatty acid oxidation. Regulatory points are numbered.

Putting Metabolic Flexibility Altogether

In the fed state, high levels of glucose, insulin, and fatty acids in the blood stream will stimulate insulin to bind to the insulin receptor causing GLUT4 and FAT/CD36 translocation to the cell membrane, allowing for glucose and fatty acid entry into the cells. Regulatory point #1 (see Figure 11.8) is where insulin gets more glucose and fatty acids into the cell. Regulatory point #2 occurs with lower levels of G6P within the cell due to increased rates of glycolysis and/or the shunting of G6P toward glycogen synthesis. Therefore, there is no allosteric inhibition on hexokinase, and glycolysis proceeds. As glycolytic flux picks up, regulatory point #3 occurs, with PFK1. As ATP needs in the cell increase due to the uptake of nutrients, ATP and citrate are at lower levels, thereby not allosterically inhibiting PFK1. At the same time, a decrease in the ATP/ADP ratio can activate PFK2, which produces fructose 2,6-bisphosphate, which allosterically activates PFK1, allowing for glycolysis to proceed, which eventually leads to an increased production of pyruvate. Next is regulatory point #4. The increase in substrate (pyruvate) will result in allosteric inhibition of pyruvate dehydrogenase kinase (PDK), thereby blocking the phosphorylation and inactivation PDH. In addition, acetyl CoA and NADH levels are not high allosterically inhibiting PDH or activating PDK, so PDH will increase the production of acetyl CoA and flux through the TCA cycle. As we accumulate ATP, NADH, and acetyl CoA, then the activity of the regulatory enzymes—HK, PFK, and PDH will slow.

At the same time glucose is entering, fatty acids are also entering FAT/CD36. But insulin is present too and this leads us to regulatory point #5 where insulin activates protein phosphatases dephosphorylating ACC and MCD. In addition, the rising levels of citrate also allosterically activate ACC2, which now becomes active, converting acetyl CoA, some of which was shuttled out of the mitochondria via the citrate shuttle (see **Figure 7.12**), to malonyl CoA. The presence of malonyl CoA then blocks CPT1, which in turn blocks fatty acid entry into the mitochondria and subsequent fatty acid oxidation. The presence of rising levels of citrate, due to increased glycolytic flux, also allosterically activate ACC2. Since fatty acids are going into the cell but not being oxidized, where do you think they are going? If you said TAG synthesis, you are correct. Recall that a fed state provokes the release of insulin, and insulin promotes the activity of anabolic pathways. TAG synthesis is an anabolic pathway and a way to store fatty acids consumed as part of a meal, for later use. A summary of regulation in a fed state that drives glucose oxidation and blocks fatty acid oxidation can be seen in Figure 11.8.

In the fasted state, the regulatory point #5 for the fed state becomes the regulatory step #1 for the fasted state. What does that mean? It means that we must relieve the inhibition of free fatty acid intake into mitochondria in order to start using free fatty acids. In a fasted state, there is an increased entry of fatty acids through fatty acid binding protein (FABP). The presence of these fatty acids, allosterically activate MCD and inhibit ACC2. When one is fasted, there is an increase in AMPK activity. While the exact mechanisms are not fully understood, it is thought that cellular decreases in glucose may contribute[4]. AMPK will phosphorylate ACC2 and MCD, thereby inhibiting ACC2 and activating MCD allowing for the conversion of malonyl CoA to acetyl CoA. This relieves the inhibition on CPT1, and fatty acids can then start to enter the mitochondria. As acetyl CoA accumulates, and NADH levels are elevated, regulatory point #2 of the fasted state occurs—namely the allosteric inhibition of PDH and allosteric activation of PDK. PDK phosphorylates PDH, further inhibiting it, reducing the conversion of pyruvate to acetyl CoA. Rising levels of ATP and citrate from fatty acid oxidation lead to regulatory point #3 in a fasted state, which means they allosterically inhibit PFK1. This slows glycolysis and will lead to the buildup of G6P, which is regulatory point #4 for a fasted state, where G6P allosterically inhibits HK, thus slowing glucose entry into glycolysis and allowing glucose to diffuse back out of cell along its concentration gradient, because it is not trapped in the cell as G6P. This regulatory process in a fasted state drives fatty acid oxidation and blocks glucose oxidation (Figure 11.9).

Metabolic Flexibility in Other Tissues

Most of what we've discussed above is really about the muscle. Insulin will increase glucose and free fatty acid uptake, glycogen synthesis, glucose oxidation, and triglyceride synthesis in the muscle. In the small intestine, glucose and fatty acids will be absorbed, and then the primary jobs of the pancreas, adipose tissue, muscle, and liver is to clear these from the circulation. Insulin is the key here—with glucose stimulation of insulin secretion, all the other pathways are put into motion. In the liver, insulin stimulates an increase in glycogenesis, blocks gluconeogenesis, inhibits fatty acid uptake, and increases TAG and cholesterol synthesis. In adipose tissue, insulin stimulates an increase in glucose and fatty acid uptake, increased glycolytic flux and glycerol production, increased TAG synthesis, and the inhibition of lipolysis. In muscle, insulin increases glucose and fatty acid uptake, glycogen synthesis, increased glycolytic flux and oxidation from glucose, and increased TAG synthesis.

What about the fasted state? Here the key molecule is glucagon. Glucagon is secreted from the pancreas when glucose levels are low. Maintenance of blood glucose levels is top priority, so glucose sparing pathways are key. There is an increase in circulating fatty acids from adipose

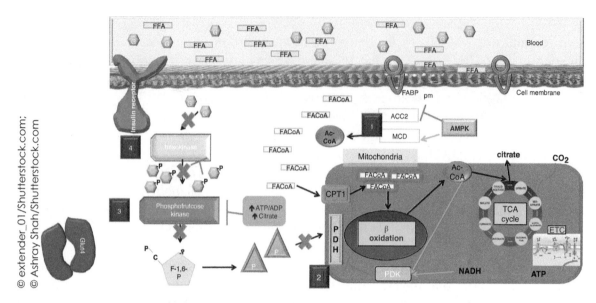

Figure 11.9: **Summary of Regulatory Factors that Drive Fatty Acid Oxidation in a Fasted State.** In a fasted state, fatty acids (FACoA) enter the cell via fatty acid binding protein-plasma membrane (FABP$_{pm}$). The build up of fatty acids into the cell allosterically activate malonyl CoA decarboxylase (MCD) and allosterically inhibit acetyl CoA carboxylase (ACC2) (Regulatory point #1). In addition rising levels of AMP can activate AMP kinase (AMPK) to phosphorylate ACC2 and MCD, activating MCD. Together, MCD converts malonyl CoA to acetyl CoA , removing the block on carnitine palmitoyl transferase (CPT1), and fatty acids can now enter. Fatty acids now proceed through beta oxidation (β-OX), increasing both acetyl CoA (Ac-CoA) and NADH levels, which allosterically inhibit pyruvate dehydrogenase (PDH) and allosterically activate pyruvate dehydrogenase kinase (PDK) (Regulatory step #2). PDK phosphorylates PDH, further inhibiting it. Pyruvate (P) can no longer be converted to Ac-CoA. The increase in ATP and citrate levels allosterically feedback and inhibit phosphofructokinase 1 (PFK1) (Regulatory step #3), so that the production of fructose 1,6-bisphosphate (F-1,6BP) decreases. With the slowing of glycolysis, glucose 6-phosphate (G6P) levels build up allosterically inhibiting hexokinase (Regulatory step #4). Hexokinase can no longer trap glucose in the cell through phosphorylation, so glucose is free to diffuse out of the cell down its concentration gradient. Regulatory points are numbered.

tissue with a rise in fatty acid oxidation in cells, sparing glucose. The liver is the key controller of blood glucose levels releasing glucose via glycogenolysis as needed. Specifically, in adipose tissue, glucagon stimulates lipolysis. In the liver, glucagon stimulates increased glycogenolysis. Increased levels of gluconeogenesis and ketogenesis will occur as needed depending on previous carbohydrate intakes and the length of the fast. Lastly in muscle, there will be an increase in fatty acid oxidation.

Metabolic Inflexibility

What is the difference between a person that would be considered *metabolically flexible*, versus one that would be considered *metabolically inflexible*? And how is this measured? And what causes the differences? These are some of the things that will be discussed in this section. Metabolic inflexibility is the inability to adjust substrate oxidation to an increase in substrate supply. In a fed state, there is an inability to increase glucose oxidation in response to increased circulating glucose levels.

In a fasted state, there is an inability to increase fatty acid oxidation in response to increased circulating fatty acid levels.

For a person that is metabolically flexible, post-prandial insulin will rise a bit, and RQ will rise a lot, and then fall as the person reaches several hours after the meal (see Figure 11.4A, adapted from Kelley and colleagues[5]). For a person that is metabolically inflexible, there tends to be a very large rise in insulin in a fed state, and a much smaller adjustment in RQ between the fed and fasted states. In a fasted state, we see that the normal situation would be a fall in total serum glucose, to a steady state, maintained first by glycogenolysis, and then from gluconeogenesis, and the RQ would fall accordingly (Figure 11.4B, adapted from Kelley and colleagues[5]). In a metabolically inflexible person, total serum glucose does not drop significantly, and the liver continues to go through glycogenolysis and gluconeogenesis. This high level of circulating glucose requires more and more insulin, eventually leading to insulin resistance. A metabolically inflexible person does not switch between glucose oxidation in a fed state and fatty acid oxidation in a fasted state, their RQ fluctuates only minimally (see Figure 11.4C, adapted from Bergouignan and colleagues[6]).

> **Terminating flexibility**
>
> What do you think? Would Arnold Schwarzenegger's character "the Terminator" be metabolically flexible or inflexible? Why?
>
>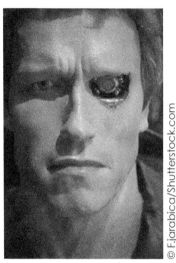
>
> © F.jarabica/Shutterstock.com

Muscle Fiber Type

Why is metabolic inflexibility present in some people and does it have to do with obesity? Some laboratories who have studied this question, have looked at the skeletal muscle, which is major contributor of glucose uptake. What they have found is that in some obese individuals, the composition of the muscle fibers is different, with more fast glycolytic fibers than slow oxidative fibers[7]. In addition, when muscle biopsies are taken from lean and obese individuals, and placed in test tubes with some palmitate, the obese individuals metabolize significantly less fat than the lean individuals[8]. From a gene expression standpoint, glycolytic enzymes are elevated in obese individuals, and fatty acid oxidation pathways are reduced, when compared to lean individuals[9]. In addition to this, fatty acids are being partitioned to tryglycerides[10], rather than being used for mitochondrial oxidation.

Insulin Resistance

Generally, the metabolically inflexible person is also insulin resistant. How do we know this? Well, there are several measures, but the gold standard is the hyperinsulinemic-euglycemic clamp procedure. In this procedure, the individual has a venous catheter inserted into each arm. One is used to infuse glucose and the other is used to infuse insulin. The dose of insulin infused is based on body size. Blood is sampled (likely from a finger prick) very frequently and glucose is infused (glucose disposal rate) to reach and maintain euglycemia. In someone who is insulin sensitive, a lot of glucose needs to be infused because they are sensitive to insulin and glucose is taken up by insulin sensitive tissues. In a person who is insulin resistant, much less glucose needs to be infused, as their tissues are not responding to insulin and taking up the glucose. The value of glucose needed to maintain euglycemia is measured in mg/kg/min and determines if someone is insulin resistant. In a normal individual, around 14 mg/kg/min of glucose would be used, compared to an obese individual who would take much less glucose to maintain euglycemia—around 8 mg/kg/min[11]. A type II diabetic would be even lower at around 5 mg/kg/min[11]. What does this mean? It means in a person who is diabetic or obese, it takes much more insulin to stimulate glucose oxidation, than in an individual who is insulin sensitive.

In addition, those who are metabolically inflexible, take longer to respond to changes in substrate oxidation when diets change. When lean subjects are placed on a high carbohydrate diet, their 24-hr RQ/RER increases to account for the greater glucose available and levels off in about 4 days[12]. When these same subjects are placed on a high-fat diet, their 24-hr RQ/RER decreases to account for greater fatty acids available and levels off in about 5 days. But for obese subjects, the change in RQ/RER is much slower and it takes an average of 6 and 8 days, respectively, to alter their RER/RQ to match fuel availability.

What comes first—does metabolic inflexibility happen first, or does insulin resistance happen first? There is evidence for both (see recent review on metabolic flexibility[13]). In fact, if you are studying metabolic inflexibility, you can quantify it as Δ in RQ = (steady state RQ – fasted RQ). A person who is metabolically flexible would have a higher Δ RQ, than someone who is metabolically inflexible. This Δ RQ can be plotted against glucose disposal rate and should be no surprise that there is a significant correlation between being metabolically inflexible and impaired insulin-stimulated glucose disposal rates[12]. Again, is it insulin resistance that is causing the metabolic inflexibility, or the other way around?

We do know that lipid accumulation in skeletal muscle is associated with insulin resistance—again though, which comes first? One thought is that there is a maximum lipid storage capacity of our adipose (both visceral and subcutaneous adipose tissue), and when adipose stores are at a maximum,

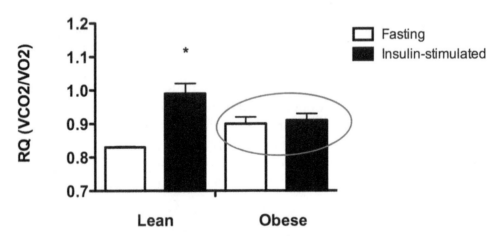

Figure 11.10: **Metabolic Inflexibility– Fasting to Fed Transition.** An RQ of 0.7 indicates oxidation of only fatty acids. An RQ of 1.0 indicates oxidation of only carbohydrates. An RQ of 0.85 indicates oxidation of 50% fatty acids and 50% carbohydrates. In a metabolically flexible person (lean), a fasted RQ would be lower than 0.85, indicating a higher level of fat oxidation, whereas in a metabolically inflexible person (obese), fasted RQ shows a greater than 0.85 value, indicating that metabolically inflexible people have higher rates of glucose oxidation over fatty acid oxidation, even in a fasted state. When stimulated with insulin and infused with glucose to reach euglycemia, a metabolically flexible person (lean) increases their RQ, showing a switch to glucose oxidation from fatty acid oxidation. A metabolically inflexible person (obese) shows no change in fuel usage upon insulin stimulation and glucose infusion to reach euglycemia.

fatty acids are diverted and if not oxidized, are stored as TAGs in other tissues, such as skeletal muscle, heart, liver, pancreas, etc. This storage of TAGs in non-adipose locations leads to lipotoxicity, or the impairment of organ function and subsequent cell death due to the presence of TAGs. Lipotoxicity eventually leads to impaired insulin signaling and eventual whole-body insulin resistance[12].

Insulin Resistance Works in Multiple Locations

In adipose tissue, if the cells are not able to respond to insulin, then lipolysis is never turned off. Remember that insulin activates phosphodiesterase (PDE) and protein phosphatases, specifically PP2, in adipose tissue. Without the stimulation of PDE to convert cAMP to AMP, cAMP continues to activate PKA and the phosphorylation of lipolysis enzymes, keeping them active. Again, without the activity of PP2, there is no dephosphorylation of the lipolysis enzymes as well (Figure 11.11). During insulin resistance, there is a constant rate of lipolysis releasing fatty acids into the blood stream, leading to high levels in circulation.

> Brush your teeth at least 2X per day
>
> For Type II Diabetes, oral health is very important as they are more prone to thrush (yeast infection in the mouth), and gum disease than those without the condition.

In the liver as well, insulin will not be able to activate PP1, which dephosphorylates glycogen synthase (making it active) and glycogen phosphorylase (making it inactive). Consequently, glycogen storage is not stimulated to store the excess glucose. At the same time, even though there are high levels of circulating glucose, glycogen phosphorylase stays on, releasing more glucose.

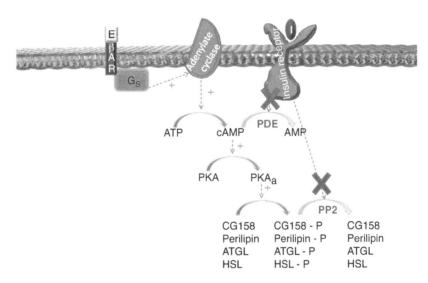

Figure 11.11: Insulin Resistance Leads to Impaired Insulin Signaling and Continued Lipolysis even in a Fed State. With metabolic inflexibility and insulin resistance, these steps (marked with an X) of insulin inhibition of lipolysis are not occurring. In a normal fed state, insulin (I) binds to the insulin receptor (IR) which leads to active phosphodiesterase (PDE), converting cAMP to AMP, blocking the PKA signaling cascade. Insulin also activates protein phosphatase 2 (PP2), which dephosphorylates lipolysis enzymes, making them inactive. Therefore, when insulin signaling is impaired, lipolysis remains on, even in a fed state, contributing to increased levels of circulating fatty acids, which can be stored ectopically leading to lipotoxicity in other organs, possibly contributing to whole body insulin resistance.

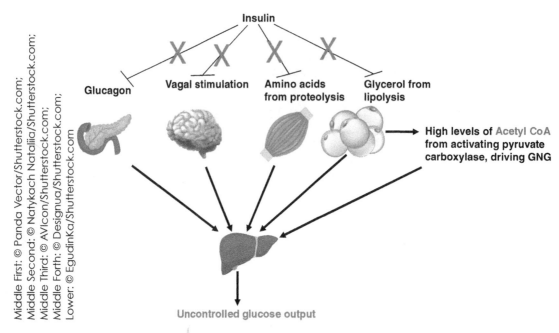

Figure 11.12: **Possible Signals by which Systemic Insulin may Regulate Hepatic Glucose Production.** During insulin resistance where insulin signalling is impaired (marked by red X), insulin can no longer block glucagon production in the pancreas, vagal stimulation of the liver, proteolysis in muscle, and lipolysis in adipose tissue. Consequently, continued glucagon and vagal stimulation, along with gluconeogenic precursors—amino acids and glycerol, and high levels of acetyl CoA from beta oxidation of fatty acids, drive glycogenolysis and gluconeogenesis in the liver, contributing to uncontrolled glucose output.

This lack of response to insulin leads to further elevated glucose levels in circulation, or hyperglycemia.

Gluconeogenesis is also less inhibited in an insulin resistant state. There is an increased presence of gluconeogenic precursors because insulin signaling no longer blocks lipolysis in adipose tissue or proteolysis in muscle[14], therefore glycerol and amino acids are available to make glucose. As insulin resistance moves into hypoinsulemia, glucagon production in the pancreas is not blocked by insulin anymore, so even in a fed state, glucagon is still in circulation[16]. Glucagon is known to stimulate gluconeogenic enzymes[17]. There is also hypothesized to be a hypothalamus (brain)—liver axis, where insulin decreases hepatic glucose production, including gluconeogenesis, in tandem with vagal stimulation. Specifically, blocking of the vagus nerve, reduces insulin's effect on the liver. One of the ways insulin normally works to suppress gluconeogenesis is through suppression of gluconeogenic enzyme transcription, specifically PEPCK and glucose-6-phosphatase[18]. Without insulin signaling to hypothalamus, there is a decrease in vagus nerve output, which would decrease insulin's affect on the liver. The vagus nerve's contribution to gluconeogenesis is still being studied. More directly, there are high levels of acetyl CoA being produced through beta oxidation. Acetyl CoA is an obligatory allosteric activator of pyruvate carboxylase, the first enzyme in the gluconeogenesis pathway. In summary, the availability of gluconeogenic precursors, the presence of glucagon,

> **Food for thought!**
>
> Stimulating the vagus nerve in humans leads to increased retention of memories[15].

the decrease in vagal stimulation, and the aberrant activity of pyruvate carboxylase all help drive gluconeogenesis, even in the presence of high circulating glucose levels[16] (Figure 11.12).

Summary

Metabolic flexibility is the ability of our body to switch between fuel sources, depending on availability. In a fed state, disposal of glucose is paramount, and a metabolically flexible person responds by ramping up glucose oxidation and decreasing fatty acid oxidation, moving their RQ/RER near 1.0. In a fasted state, it is paramount to spare blood glucose, and a metabolically flexible person responds by ramping up fatty acid oxidation and decreasing glucose oxidation, moving their RER/RQ closer to 0.7. Our body's ability to do this is called the glucose-fatty acid cycle, or Randle cycle. Allosteric and covalent regulation on these key enzymes: hexokinase, phosphofructokinase, pyruvate dehydrogenase, acetyl CoA carboxylase, and malonyl CoA decarboxylase, allow the glucose-fatty acid cycle to function.

A metabolically inflexible person cannot respond to changes in fuel availability, maintaining an RQ/RER near 0.9, preferentially oxidizing glucose, even in the presence of high circulating fatty acids. Metabolically inflexible people have a higher composition of fast glycolytic muscle fibers that rely more on anaerobic metabolism and have a higher ratio of glycolytic enzymes as compared to oxidative enzymes. The answer to whether metabolic inflexibility leads to insulin resistance or vice versus, is unknown. What is known, is that in the absence of proper insulin signaling, lipolysis proceeds unregulated, leading to high circulating free fatty acids. In addition, glycogenolysis cannot be turned off and gluconeogenesis gets activated in direct and indirect ways, both leading to increased levels of hepatic glucose production, contributing to even higher levels of circulating glucose. Lastly, the pancreas continues to make glucagon due to hypoinsulemia, which further drives glycogenolysis and lipolysis.

Points to Ponder

➣ Trace the glucose-fatty acid cycle starting with insulin in a fed state, leading to the blocking of CPT1. How is ATP generated, what is the substrate and what are the steps? Now trace the glucose-fatty acid cycle starting with fatty acids, leading to the blocking of PDH, PFK1, and HK. Now, how is ATP generated, what is the substrate and what are the steps?

➣ Can one be metabolically inflexible in the absence of obesity? Why or why not?

➣ Search "What leads to insulin resistance?" What are some of the theories presented? Do they mention metabolic flexibility?

➣ Obese research participants have been found to have more fast glycolytic muscle fibers, than slow oxidative fibers. We know that genetics determines muscle fiber type, with some ability for fiber type switching. Do you think that those who are born with more of the fast glycolytic fibers are predestined for obesity? If so, then how about world-class sprinters who also have a high level of fast glycolytic fibers?

References

1. Randle PJ, Garland PB, Hales CN, Newsholme EA. The glucose fatty-acid cycle. Its role in insulin sensitivity and the metabolic disturbances of diabetes mellitus. *Lancet.* 1963;1(7285):785–789.

2. Hue L, Taegtmeyer H. The Randle cycle revisited: a new head for an old hat. *Am J Physiol Endocrinol Metab.* 2009;297(3):E578–591.

3. Saha AK, Schwarsin AJ, Roduit R, et al. Activation of malonyl-CoA decarboxylase in rat skeletal muscle by contraction and the AMP-activated protein kinase activator 5-aminoimidazole-4-carboxamide-1-beta-D-ribofuranoside. *J Biol Chem.* 2000;275(32):24279–24283.

4. Canto C, Jiang LQ, Deshmukh AS, et al. Interdependence of AMPK and SIRT1 for metabolic adaptation to fasting and exercise in skeletal muscle. *Cell Metab.* 2010;11(3):213–219.

5. Kelley DE, Goodpaster B, Wing RR, Simoneau JA. Skeletal muscle fatty acid metabolism in association with insulin resistance, obesity, and weight loss. *Am J Physiol.* 1999;277(6 Pt 1):E1130–1141.

6. Bergouignan A, Antoun E, Momken I, et al. Effect of contrasted levels of habitual physical activity on metabolic flexibility. *J Appl Physiol (1985).* 2013;114(3):371–379.

7. Tanner CJ, Barakat HA, Dohm GL, et al. Muscle fiber type is associated with obesity and weight loss. *Am J Physiol Endocrinol Metab.* 2002;282(6):E1191–1196.

8. Kim JY, Hickner RC, Cortright RL, Dohm GL, Houmard JA. Lipid oxidation is reduced in obese human skeletal muscle. *Am J Physiol Endocrinol Metab.* 2000;279(5):E1039–1044.

9. Simoneau JA, Kelley DE. Altered glycolytic and oxidative capacities of skeletal muscle contribute to insulin resistance in NIDDM. *J Appl Physiol (1985).* 1997;83(1):166–171.

10. Hulver MW, Berggren JR, Carper MJ, et al. Elevated stearoyl-CoA desaturase-1 expression in skeletal muscle contributes to abnormal fatty acid partitioning in obese humans. *Cell Metab.* 2005;2(4):251–261.

11. Nadeau KJ, Maahs DM, Daniels SR, Eckel RH. Childhood obesity and cardiovascular disease: links and prevention strategies. *Nat Rev Cardiol.* 2011;8(9):513–525.

12. Galgani JE, Moro C, Ravussin E. Metabolic flexibility and insulin resistance. *Am J Physiol Endocrinol Metab.* 2008;295(5):E1009–1017.

13. Goodpaster BH, Sparks LM. Metabolic Flexibility in Health and Disease. *Cell Metab.* 2017;25(5):1027–1036.

14. Wang X, Hu Z, Hu J, Du J, Mitch WE. Insulin resistance accelerates muscle protein degradation: Activation of the ubiquitin-proteasome pathway by defects in muscle cell signaling. *Endocrinology.* 2006;147(9):4160–4168.

15. Ghacibeh GA, Shenker JI, Shenal B, Uthman BM, Heilman KM. The influence of vagus nerve stimulation on memory. *Cogn Behav Neurol.* 2006;19(3):119–122.

16. Girard J. The inhibitory effects of insulin on hepatic glucose production are both direct and indirect. *Diabetes.* 2006;55(Supplement 2):S65–S69.

17. Granner D, Pilkis S. The genes of hepatic glucose metabolism. *J Biol Chem.* 1990;265(18):10173–10176.

18. Inoue H, Ogawa W, Asakawa A, et al. Role of hepatic STAT3 in brain-insulin action on hepatic glucose production. *Cell Metab.* 2006;3(4):267–275.

CHAPTER 12

Let's Exercise

Do you exercise? Do you get the recommended amounts of exercise? Why? Or why not? What *are* the recommended amounts of exercise? The 2008 physical activity guidelines state that adults should get 150 min of moderate intensity exercise a week, or 75 min of vigorous intensity exercise a week, or a combination of the two. In addition, an adult should do strength training exercises 2–3 times a week. Did you know that in a recent survey, only 2.4% of Americans knew the correct guideline[1]? Wow! In addition, a cross-sectional study showed that fewer than 10% of American adults met the physical activity guidelines, as measured by wearing an accelerometer[2]. Our society has some work to do. The importance of exercise cannot be underscored. In fact, as we'll find out in this chapter, *most metabolic issues can be fixed with exercise*. Really? Yes! Let's figure out why and how.

> ### Incoming...
> The 2018 Physical Activity Guidelines are due to be released soon—but likely after this text is published. A draft of the guidelines which are open for comments can be found at: https://health.gov/paguidelines/second-edition/report.aspx

As discussed in chapter 11, metabolic flexibility is the body's ability to switch between different substrates for energy, based on substrate availability. This inability to metabolically adapt is commonly observed in overweight and obese individuals, who preferentially store fat, versus oxidize it for energy[3]–not very metabolically flexible. One of the places that fat gets stored is within muscle (intramuscular TAGs—IMTGs), and this storage is linked with insulin resistance[3]. Insulin resistance is defined as the decreased ability of cells to respond to the action of insulin in transporting glucose from the bloodstream into muscle and adipose tissue.

> ### Body Mass Index (BMI)
> Body mass index is a common weight standard derived from the ratio of a person's height to their weight. Based on population standards, one is categorized as overweight if their BMI is greater or equal to 25 kg/m^2 and categorized as obese if their BMI is greater or equal to 30 kg/m^2.

While IMTGs do not directly cause insulin resistance, it is known that the intermediates of TAG synthesis, diacylglycerols (DAGs) and fatty acyl CoAs, can interfere with insulin signaling if left to accumulate. Weight loss does reduce IMTGs and improves insulin sensitivity, but does not change rates of fatty acid oxidation[3]. Exercise on the other hand, even without weight loss, not only increases insulin sensitivity, but also increases fatty acid metabolism[3]. In fact, participants who have gastric bypass see improvements in insulin sensitivity, but those that add in exercise on top of the weight loss get a significantly greater improvement in insulin sensitivity[4]. The importance of exercise in relationship to our body's healthy metabolism cannot be underestimated.

So, for those wanting to improve their health and lose weight, the adage to lose weight says, "Eat less; move more." While calorie cutting is important, the combination of weight loss and exercise together show a greater success in the context of health outcomes because independently they both have beneficial effects. Exercise on its own is known to contribute to cardio metabolic wellness and improve cognitive performance[5]. In addition, it is important in the prevention and maintenance of diseases including cancer, cardiovascular disease, diabetes, neurological diseases, and osteoporosis[5]. While weight loss alone has been shown to improve hypertension, coronary artery disease, stroke, diabetes, dyslipidemia, non-alcoholic fatty liver, gall-stones, sleep apnea, asthma, fertility, cancer prevention and mortality, and mental health[6]. The list seems to go on and on. Although physical activity has been shown only to have a modest effect ($< 3\%$) on weight loss alone, it has an additive effect when combined with reduced calorie intake. In combination, exercise and reduced calorie intake have been shown to minimize weight regain[7].

The National Weight Control Registry catalogs people who have lost 30 lbs or more and maintained that weight loss for at least one year[8]. One of the major characteristics of those that are on the registry is their physical activity habits. The average woman reported burning 2545 kcal/week in physical activity, and the average man reported burning an average of 3293 kcal/week. This equates to approximately 400+ min of moderate intensity exercise per week, by far exceeding the physical activity guidelines. The importance of exercise in weight maintenance is crucial. Those dieters who do not exercise, are basically not on the registry because weight loss has not been maintained.

Energy Systems During Exercise

So why is exercise so crucial to our metabolic health and weight maintenance? Let's start by talking about skeletal muscle physiology, and the available energy systems. We have three energy systems available for skeletal muscle cells to use—these systems keep ATP levels at or very close to the levels that are found at rest. No one system works by itself, but all work in tandem, with one system dominating.

Creatine Phosphate

First, there is the creatine phosphate system. Remember that this system regenerates ATP (from ADP) by hydrolyzing creatine phosphate. However, this system is really only for bursts of energy for very short periods of time or at the very start of exercise, and dominates for about 10–15 seconds at most. Sprinters, weight-lifters, shot-putters, etc. rely heavily on this system. In fact, the concentration of creatine phosphate in muscle is higher in fast glycolytic muscle fibers over slow oxidative fibers. Recall from earlier (Chapter 9) creatine is a nitrogen-containing compound that is synthesized in the liver. Creatine can also be taken as a supplement and there is evidence that creatine supplementation can improve muscular performance in high-intensity resistance exercises[9].

Ponder this

Creatine isn't a protein, but it is derived from amino acids. Do you remember which ones? Check back to Chapter 9 if you don't and make sure you do!

creatine

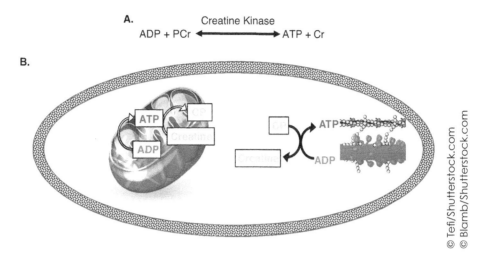

A.

Creatine Kinase

ADP + PCr ⟷ ATP + Cr

B.

© Tefi/Shutterstock.com
© Blamb/Shutterstock.com

Figure 12.1: **Creatine Phosphate System. (A)** Creatine kinase (CK) works in both directions, adding a phosphate onto creatine (C), making creatine phosphate (CP), a cellular storage of energy or catalyzes the addition of that phosphate from creatine to ADP to make ATP, to continue muscular work. **(B)** CK is located in multiple areas in the cell. In the mitochondria, where ATP is plenty CK, adds a phosphate to C, making CP. Near actin and myosin, CK removes the phosphate from CP, making ATP from ADP.

Endogenous creatine is released into blood from the liver, and cells like muscle that have creatine transporters, take up creatine for use in the cell. The creatine then diffuses to places in the cell (found both in the mitochondria and the cytoplasm) where creatine kinase enzymes are found and ATP is being produced or used. Creatine kinase catalyzes the reaction, which results in the transfer of a phosphate group from ATP to creatine, producing creatine phosphate (Figure 12.1). The stored phosphocreatine is ready to regenerate that ATP when it is needed. How is this done—creatine kinase works in both directions. Cytoplasmic creatine kinase removes the phosphate from creatine phosphate and adds it to ADP, making ATP. ATP can now continue to cock that myosin head for muscular contraction or be used for other ATPases. Mitochondrial creatine kinase adds a phosphate from ATP that is being generated in the electron transport chain to creatine, producing creatine phosphate for future use.

Anaerobic Glycolysis

As soon as glucose begins to be released from glycogen, anaerobic glycolysis, our second system, is activated. When the phosphocreatine levels drop and glucose starts to become more available, either from glycogenolysis or from the blood, anaerobic glycolysis becomes the predominant energy system. This system, as you hopefully recall, produces lactate from glucose. The primary source of glucose for muscle metabolism is stored muscle glycogen. When glucose is released from glycogen; it is released as glucose-1-phosphate (G1P). G1P is isomerized to glucose-6-phosphate (G6P), which skips hexokinase (HK), and enters in at the second step of glycolysis. Because G6P skips the step requiring HK, investment of 1 ATP is spared. Consequently, when glucose comes from glycogen, the net ATP yield of glycolysis is 3 ATP (see Figure 12.2). However, like the creatine phosphate system, anaerobic glycolysis cannot be sustained for very long, and only gives about 2—3 minutes of energy availability when exercising maximally. Those running the 400M or swimming the 100M fly, would benefit from anaerobic glycolytic activity.

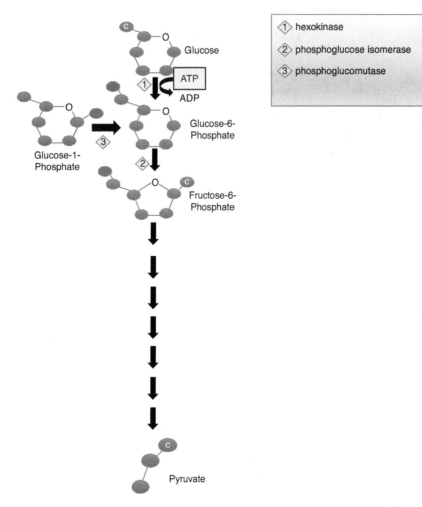

Figure 12.2: **Glucose from Glycogen Entering Glycolysis in Muscle.** Glucose is released from glycogen as glucose-1-phosphate (G1P), which isomerizes to glucose-6-P (G6P), via phosphoglucomutase, and can now enter glycolysis, skipping the first enzymatic step of hexokinase. Since the first step is skipped that involves the investment of 1 ATP, the net ATP yield from glycolysis with glucose from glycogen is 3 ATP, versus 2 ATP from blood glucose.

Oxidative Phosphorylation

Finally, we have oxidative phosphorylation. This third system cannot produce ATP as quickly but can do so for a long period. Oxidative phosphorylation is the sustainable system for ATP production in exercise that lasts longer than 2–3 minutes. This system can use both glucose and fatty acids (and amino acids and ketones if available) as substrates. It is worth noting here, that oxidative phosphorylation rate is not the limiting factor in ATP generation, but the ability of our body to pump oxygen-rich blood to working muscle and to have that oxygen transferred to the mitochondria. Factors that can affect oxygen getting to the electron transport chain include:

1. Pulmonary ventilation- how much air we can get in
2. Oxygenation of hemoglobin- how much oxygen we can carry
3. Release of oxygen from hemoglobin- how much oxygen we can unload
4. Capillarization at the muscle level- how close can we get the oxygen to each muscle fiber
5. Ability for muscle to use oxygen- the number of mitochondria, oxidative enzymes, myoglobin, etc.

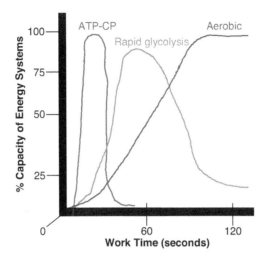

Figure 12.3: **Energy Systems During Exercise.** ATP reserves in the cell are used up immediately at the start of exercise, to keep muscle contraction going, the creatine phosphate (CP) system responds first, donating phosphates to ADP, making ATP. It, however, is exhausted in about 10–15 sec. As the CP system runs out of phosphates, anaerobic glycolysis picks up producing ATP and lactate. This high level of glycolysis can only be maintained for about 2–3 min. During the first 0–3 min, aerobic oxidation phosphorylation is increasing its contribution to ATP generation, and will be the dominant energy system used for the remainder of exercise.

Take a look at Figure 12.3. As working time increases from 0 seconds to 5 minutes, you can see the initial burst of energy that comes from the creatine phosphate system, then a ramp up of anaerobic glycolysis, and finally an increase in oxidative phosphorylation that is sustained over the duration of exercise. Again, all three systems are always working to produce ATP, time dictates which system is the dominant system.

Fuel Sources During Exercise

Where does the energy come from for anaerobic glycolysis or oxidative phosphorylation? There are five primary sources of fuel to choose from: muscle glycogen, plasma glucose, plasma fatty acids, intramuscular TAGs (IMTGs), and amino acids. Which one of these will be used and when? How do you maximize your fuel stores? Should athletes pre-load on carbohydrates, fat, or protein? Do glycogen stores need to be high prior to exercise? How would a low carbohydrate diet affect fuel sources? Some of the answers to these questions can be figured out if one knows more about the specific exercise and the individual athlete. What is the intensity and duration of the exercise that is being done? How trained is the athlete? What is their level of glycogen stores? Are they supplementing with an energy source during the exercise? Let's look at some of the different conditions and determine what fuel should (and will) be selected.

Low Intensity Exercise

We discussed VO_2 max in Chapter 11, but if the concept is still confusing, think about it as effort level. If someone is at 100% VO_2 max, they are giving their maximum effort. When a person walks at low intensity, which would be equivalent to 25–30% VO_2 max, IMTGs and plasma fatty acids are the predominate substrates with a small contribution of glucose. Really, a person doing low intensity exercise doesn't change the fuel source from what they would be using under rest, as there isn't a significant energy demand. Does this change whether the person is in a fed or in a fasted state? Not really, although, as you know, in the fasted state, more lipolysis is occurring, and so plasma fatty acid availability will be even higher. Fat is favored in fact, for low-moderate intensity exercises <50% of VO_2 max.

High Intensity Exercise

What happens when the intensity of exercise goes up to 85% of VO_2 max? Blood flow to skeletal muscle increases, but this means that blood flow to other organs decreases. Adipose tissue is not going to have as much blood flow, and therefore while lipolysis continues, fatty acids are not released and transported to the muscle. What happens then? Substrate selection must change back to glucose as the preferred substrate. Fat cannot be oxidized at sufficient rates to meet ATP demand as intensity increases, so at about 50–65% VO_2 max, 50% of energy yield is from carbohydrates. The reasons that fat oxidation can't keep up are due to a couple factors. Fatty acid transfer into mitochondria is slow—remember the carnitine shuttle—and more oxygen is needed to metabolize fat than is needed for carbohydrates. So, as intensity increases, muscle increases uptake of glucose, dropping blood glucose levels during exercise. Glucose uptake by muscle during exercise is not insulin-independent, and rather dependent on contraction intensity. So, why don't we see hypoglycemia at 100% VO_2 max? Because the liver keeps supplying glucose via glycogenolysis and/or gluconeogenesis. And since, blood flow is directed to the muscle tissue, the glucose that is released by the liver can quickly get there. Muscle glycogen can also contribute to muscle glucose for energy, but those stores are much lower than what is found in the liver.

> **Energy Drinks**
>
> Energy drinks contain a lot of caffeine and many contain sugar. The energy burst is short-lived and some can cause a "crash" afterwards. Consumer Reports measured the caffeine content in 27 of the most top-selling brands, with 5-hour energy having the highest caffeine level at 242 mg/serving (an 8 oz cup of coffee contains 100mg). Check out: https://www.consumerreports.org/cro/magazine/2012/12/the-buzz-on-energy-drink-caffeine/index.htm for all beverages. Remember to limit caffeine to a maximum of 400 mg/day.

The Crossover Effect

The term "the crossover effect" was coined by Brooks and Mercier in 1994[10], and refers to the switching of substrates as intensity of exercise increases. At rest, and up to about 50–65% intensity of VO_2 max (after 20 min of exercise), fat is going to be the preferred substrate, but as intensity increases, the contribution of carbohydrates increases, and the contribution of fats begin to decrease. At the 50–65% mark, the "crossover" occurs, where fat and carbohydrate utilization are both at about 50% or equal to each other (Figure 12.4). As the intensity increases above 50–65%, carbohydrates contribute more and more to ATP generation. In an untrained person, the cross-over point might be closer to 50%, where in trained athletes, the crossover point shifts to perhaps 70 or 75% before carbohydrates become the predominate substrate. This shift to the right with training, spares glycogen and blood glucose and accounts for training-induced increases in endurance for prolonged exercise.

What contributes to this? Remember as mentioned earlier, as intensity increases, blood shifts away from adipose tissue, fatty acid transfer into the mitochondria is slow, and more oxygen is need for fatty acid oxidation. In fact, glycogenolysis and glycolysis can produce acetyl CoA at a faster

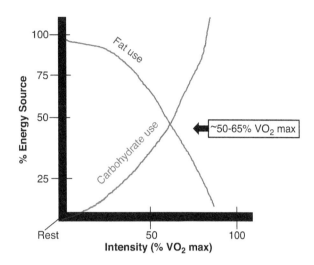

Figure 12.4: **The Cross-Over Effect.** At rest and at low to moderate intensity exercise, after ~20min when fatty acids become available, fatty acid oxidation will dominate, as we have ample stores and the ATP produced from each fatty acid can be upwards of 4x the amount of a molecule of glucose. However, as intensity of exercise increases, fatty acid oxidation can not keep up with the ATP demand and glucose oxidation starts to play a bigger role. At about 50–65% VO_2 max (or intensity level), there is an equal contribution of fatty acids and glucose for oxidation. This is the cross-over point. After this point, glucose oxidation rates will increase with fatty acid oxidation rates decreasing. Untrained individuals have a cross-over point closer to 50%, with highly trained athletes having a cross-over point exceeding 65%, which allows them to oxidize fatty acids a lot longer.

rate than beta oxidation. So, if ATP cannot be generated at high enough rates from fatty acid oxidation to meet intensity, then we must swap fuels. To meet energy demands, glucose from glycogen is released for oxidation. But what causes glycogenolysis? The sympatho-adrenal response, of course!. The sympathetic nervous system is half of our autonomic nervous system (the other being the parasympathetic), which controls our involuntary nervous system, like heart rate, vasoconstriction/vasodilation, digestive movements, etc. Unlike the parasympathetic nervous system, which is our rest and digest half, the sympathetic nervous system (SNS) is our fight or flight. Stimulation of the SNS slows peristalsis in the digestive system, causes pupil dilation, leads to bronchodilation in the lung, and increased heart rate and force of contraction of the heart, all outcomes that we see with exercise. The SNS has three possible paths for sympathetic nerves—the sympathetic chain ganglion, the collateral ganglion and the middle of the adrenal gland, or adrenal medulla. Sympathetic stimulation of the adrenal medulla causes the release of circulating catecholamines, such as epinephrine (E) and norepinephrine (NE). During exercise, the SNS is stimulated to respond to the stresses on the body and can stimulate the release of catecholamines, which can bind to muscle fibers and initiate the glycogenolysis signaling pathway (see **Figure 10.3**). Catecholamines also stimulate lipolysis. Think about an untrained person—their "stress response" to intense exercise will cause the release of catecholamines early on into the onset of exercise, stimulating the switch to carbohydrates. In a trained person, intense exercise is going to be less of a stressor, and so the switch can be delayed.

Another contributor to the crossover effect is the amount of lactate that is released. As glycogenolysis ramps up, glycolysis flux will be increased, which will lead to increased lactate production. Lactate can stimulate GPR81, a G-coupled protein receptor exclusively expressed on adipocytes, which can downregulate adenylate cyclase, reducing the formation of cAMP, and subsequent downregulation of lipolysis[11] (Figure 12.5). Again, the trained athlete is going to (at least initially) release

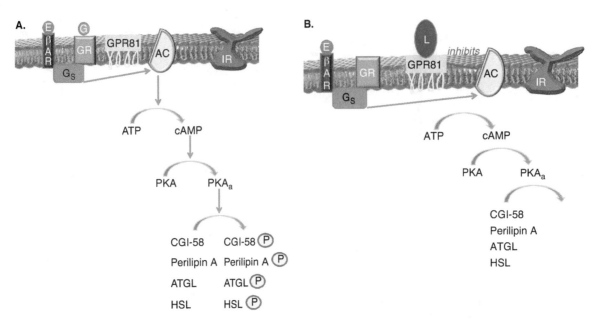

Figure 12.5: **Inhibition of Lipolysis through Lactate Binding to GPR81 on Adipocytes. (A)** Under circumstances when lactate is absent, epinephrine (E) or glucagon (G), will bind to its receptor activating adenylate cyclase (AC), which coverts ATP to cAMP, which then activates protein kinase A (PKA). PKA phosphorylates the lipolytic enzymes, making them active and increasing lipolysis. **(B)** GPR81 is a G-coupled protein found exclusively on adipocytes. When lactate binds, it blocks adenylate cyclase (AC) from converting ATP to cAMP, thereby blocking the activation of PKA and the subsequent phosphorylation of lipolytic enzymes, decreasing lipolysis in adipocytes. This process contributes to the fuel selection of glucose oxidation at high intensities.

less lactate than the untrained person, so again, this would delay the reduction in lipolysis, compared to an untrained person.

   We cannot end this section without mentioning that it takes about 20 min for fatty acids to become a major contributor to ATP generation. At the beginning of exercise, glucose oxidation will dominate, as glycogenolysis is stimulated and glucose is readily available. It takes time to stimulate lipolysis, transport the free fatty acids in blood, uptake them by the muscle cell, and get them into the mitochondria for beta oxidation. So, in the cross-over model, a person would need to be exercising about 20 min at low to moderate intensity to see fatty acids as the major fuel source.

Physiological Adaptations to Exercise Training

Glycogen

We all know that over time, as we exercise, we get better at it. What is it that makes exercise easier? What are the physical adaptations to the body due to exercise training? One adaptation is the quantity of glycogen stores, which are significantly increased with training[12]. The amount of starting glycogen that a person has also determines how long they can exercise prior to fatigue, especially with high intensity exercise. In fact, glycogen depletion is the single most consistent observation that correlates with fatigue. A study done by Spencer et al. (1992), took subjects and had them exercise at 75% VO$_2$ max on a cycle ergometer on two separate occasions for the same time period[13]. The first occasion, the muscle glycogen levels were low (LG), due to previous exercise and a low carbohydrate diet. On the second occasion, subjects rested and ate a high carbohydrate (HG) for three days preceding the test. The larger glycogen content, the more it was used. There was a change of 175 mmol glucosyl units/kg dry wt (that is to say the amount of glucose units from glycogen found per weight of a muscle sample that has been dried) in the LG group compared to 372 mmol glucosyl units/kg dry wt in the HG group. Glycogen can also be broken down anaerobically, where fat oxidation cannot. The HG condition had a significantly higher circulation of blood lactate, pointing to the use of anaerobic metabolism, whereas the LG condition had a significantly higher heart rate and VO$_2$, trying to get oxygen to working muscle for fat oxidation.

Mitochondria, Oxidative Enzymes, Capillarization, and Muscle Fiber Type

Other improvements with exercise training include increased number of mitochondria in muscle—so an actual increase in mitochondrial biogenesis[14]. Along with the number of mitochondria, comes an increase in mitochondrial oxidative enzymes. In fact with moderate training (30–60 min at 70–80% of VO$_2$ max, 3–5 times weekly), muscles can display a 40–50% increase in these oxidative enzymes with trained athletes having 3–4 times more oxidative enzyme levels than non-athletes[15]. Again, with moderate training, capillarization of skeletal muscle may increase by 50% and trained athletes have 2–3 times more capillaries per muscle fiber than non-athletes[15].

We talked in chapter 11 about different muscle fiber types, mainly fast glycolytic and slow oxidative. Fast glycolytic, sometimes called white muscle, has a low mitochondrial content, low capillarization, and is high in glycolytic enzymes. It is the perfect muscle type for quick bursts of activities. Slow oxidative, sometimes called red muscle, has a high mitochondrial content, high level of capillarization and myoglobin (giving it a red appearance), and a high content of oxidative enzymes. There is another muscle fiber that has a combination of features of the two, and not surprisingly is called fast oxidative glycolytic (FOG). With aerobic training, there can be fiber type switching from fast glycolytic to fast oxidative glycolytic and some slow oxidative, increasing these aerobic fibers. This makes sense because these are the types of muscle fibers that have more mitochondria and are associated with endurance.

Other Adaptations to Exercise

Did you know that highly-trained athletes store intramuscular triglycerides (IMTGs) similarly to those in an obese state? In fact, both endurance trained participants and obese participants have similar levels of IMTGs, both of which are significantly greater than lean controls[16]. But unlike the ectopic fat storage of obesity, IMTGs in muscle allow athletes to reduce the time it takes to rely on fat oxidation (remember the 20 minutes?), using IMTGs more so than plasma fatty acids. In addition, after exercise rates of lipolysis are greater in trained person than an untrained person to replenish these IMTGs, to be able to use the next time.

Heart and lungs also have increased capacity. In the lungs, there is an increase in blood flow and surface for gas exchange, as well as an increase in tidal volume[17]. In the heart, there is an increase in myocardium (or the cardiac muscle itself), which also leads to a lower resting heart rate in trained athletes[17]. Systemically there is a general increase in blood volume, the number of red blood cells, and overall capillary density[17]. Blood pressure is also improved, making exercise a crucial component for those who are pre-hypertensive or hypertensive[18]. In fact, you would be hard-pressed to find a body system that won't improve with response to exercise.

Detraining

All these adaptations to exercise are wonderful, but many are lost when one's exercise routine concludes. The oxidative enzyme increases mentioned earlier, occur over 6–8 weeks of time. When training stops, these increases are lost within 4–6 weeks, which is faster than declines seen in capillarization and VO_2 max[15]. As mentioned earlier, mitochondrial content can increase, and in fact after about 4–5 weeks of training, mitochondrial numbers can double[19]. However, in just one week of detraining, 50% of this increase is lost and after 5 weeks of detraining all the adaptation is lost, with retraining taking another 4 weeks to gain it back[19].

> **The word: Detraining**
>
> If you search the dictionary, the definition of detraining is the action of leaving a train. Researchers use the word to mean, the cessation of exercise. A quick Pubmed search shows the first article using the word detraining was in 1965[20] and the first review article referring to detraining was published in 1989[21].

In a pivotal study by Booth, F. in 1977, mitochondrial numbers via the protein cytochrome c, were estimated based on the protein half-life[22]. If a trained athlete were to be "injured" and unable to exercise for a week, a 50% decrease in muscle mitochondrial levels is estimated, and due to the protein degradation rate and the synthesis rate for new mitochondria, it would take the athlete about 3–4 weeks of re-training to recover from the week off. That is disheartening news.

Hormones

Several hormones play a role during exercise. Epinephrine suppresses insulin release from the pancreas. Remember insulin drives anabolic pathways and during exercise, we are in a catabolic state. Instead, glucagon and catecholamines are in circulation driving those catabolic pathways. Growth hormone levels go up, which also help to stimulate lipolysis and fat oxidation. Lastly, exercise is a stress on the body, so levels of cortisol increase, which stimulate protein breakdown—more on that later on.

> **Exercise and metabolic disease**
>
> In individuals with insulin resistance, exercise can help to increase glucose uptake through an alternate GLUT4 translocation method—calcium released during muscle contraction[23].

If insulin is suppressed and skeletal muscle is dependent on some level of glucose oxidation depending on intensity, and glycogen levels are decreasing within the muscle, how will glucose get into the muscle cell? There is an alternative way for GLUT4 translocation, independent of insulin. In contracting muscles, the sarcoplasmic reticulum releases calcium for purpose of stimulating muscle contraction. This calcium can also stimulate a separate set of GLUT4 transporters, that are calcium sensitive, allowing for translocation.

The neat thing about exercise is that even after a bout of exercise, when muscle glycogen stores are depleted, glucose uptake is facilitated–without an increase in insulin. Exercise is so important for diabetics! In addition, muscle is more insulin-sensitive than in a resting state. This insulin-sensitivity will persist for several hours, with fatty acids being the preferred fuel source, preserving glucose use for glycogen replenishment. While this is a transient effect, oxidizing fat post-exercise is always a plus. In fact, many people believe that they need to be oxidizing fat during exercise to lose weight. Remember the intensity in which fat oxidation dominates? Low-intensity, right? If instead one exercised at a higher intensity using glucose oxidation, fat oxidation will still occur, but at the conclusion of exercise, when glycogen is being replenished. Remember, you can burn more calories with higher intensity exercise. Don't be fooled by the "fat-burning" zone on the aerobic machines at the gym.

Amino Acids as Energy Sources During Exercise

We have spent the bulk of the time talking about glucose and fatty acid oxidation. But yes, muscle protein can be used as fuel source, however this usually only happens with prolonged exercise or in situations where the glycogen stores are either depleted or very limited when the exercise started. Out of all 20 amino acids, which are most important? Branched chain amino acids. The backbones of branched chain amino acids (remember, these are leucine, isoleucine, and valine) can be used immediately to make ATP. Leucine catabolism produces an acetyl CoA and an acetoacetate, isoleucine produces an acetyl CoA and a propinoyl CoA, and valine produces a propinoyl CoA and a CO_2. Remember propinoyl CoA from odd-chained fatty acid oxidation? It can be converted to succinyl CoA. Regardless, all feed into the TCA cycle, making ATP. These branched chain amino acids (BCAA) make up 35–40% of the essential amino acids in dietary proteins, and up to 18% of proteins in skeletal muscles. Muscle also expresses more of the branched chain aminotransferase (BCAT) enzyme than other tissues such as the liver, and this enables muscle to utilize the BCAAs in metabolism.

BCAT is the first enzymatic step in the catabolism of BCAAs, utilizing alpha ketoglutarate, and forming branched chain keto acids and glutamate (Figure 12.6). Glutamate is a vital amino acid in

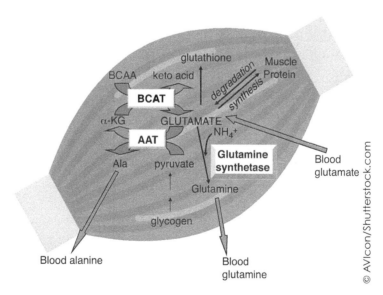

Figure 12.6: **Skeletal Branched Chain Amino Acid (BCAA) Metabolism.** During protein degradation, BCAA amino acids are favored for energy catabolism, due to the availability of their carbon skeletons. BCAAs plus alpha ketoglutarate (α-KG) are converted to a keto acid and glutamate via the enzyme branched chain amino transferase (BCAT) . Glutamate has several fates. It can be combined with pyruvate (coming from glycolysis) via amino acid transferase (AAT) to form α-KG and alanine. Alanine can leave the muscle for gluconeogenesis in the muscle. Glutamate can help with nitrogen removal in the muscle by accepting an ammonium ion (NH_4^+) via glutamate synthase. (Blood glutamate can also be absorbed and used in this fashion too.) Glutamate can be used as the precursor to glutathione, an important molecule for mediating reactive oxygen species (ROS). Glutamate can also be used as a needed amino acid during regular protein synthesis.

clearing nitrogen from muscle cells, as it can accept an ammonium ion (NH_4^+) and via the enzyme glutamine synthetase, produce the amino acid, glutamine. If not making glutamine, the glutamate can immediately be used with pyruvate (from glycolysis) to produce alpha-ketoglutarate and alanine, via alanine aminotransferase (AAT). You may recognize alanine from our talks on gluconeogenesis. Alanine, because of its ability to be converted back into pyruvate in one enzymatic step, is an important gluconeogenic precursor for the liver. Alanine produced by AAT in skeletal muscle, can leave the cell and then be picked up by the liver (Figure 12.6). Here is another reason why BCAA catabolism is the most important amino acid catabolism in metabolism.

The second enzymatic step in BCAA catabolism, which is also the regulatory point in the process, is branched chain keto acid dehydrogenase (BCKAD). BCKAD catalyzes the irreversible oxidative decarboxylation reaction of the BCAAs. Like many other enzymes we have looked at, BCKAD is regulated both covalently and allosterically. BCKAD is active when dephosphorylated, so BCKAD phosphatase is crucial for this. On the other hand, BCKAD kinase, phosphorylates BCKAD, inhibiting it (Figure 12.7). BCKAD is also allosterically inhibited by the three products of BCKAD (one product for each BCAA)—isovaleryl CoA, α-methylbutyryl CoA, and isobutyryl CoA. In addition, hormones can also play a role. Insulin stimulates BCKAD kinase (decreasing BCAA catabolism), such that in someone with poorly controlled diabetes, BCAA catabolism would proceed, due to insulin resistance. Conversely, BCKAD kinase is inhibited allosterically by the substrate for leucine catabolism-α-ketoisocaproate, driving BCAA catabolism. In addition, cortisol decreases BCKAD kinase activity (increasing BCAA catabolism), so in cases of starvation or prolonged exercise that produce stress on the body, cortisol is working to break down BCAAs for their carbon skeleton, as well as for glutamate production.

Last to consider during BCAA catabolism is the fate of glutamate. We mentioned that it can be used to make alanine and that it can also be used to pick up an ammonium ion and form glutamine. Glutamine can be picked up in the liver and deaminated via the enzyme glutaminase, sending the

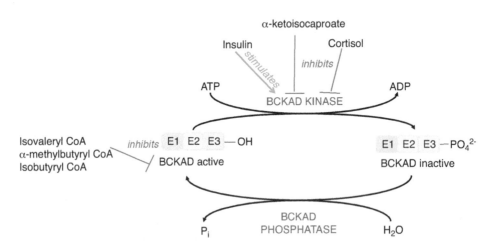

Figure 12.7: **Regulation of Branched Chain Keto Acid Dehydrogenase (BCKAD).** BCKAD in its active form is dephosphorylated. This is facilitated by BCKAD phosphatase. BCKAD is inactive when phosphorylated by BCKAD kinase. BCKAD is also allosterically inhibited by the 3 products of the enzyme—isovaleryl CoA, α-methylbutyryl CoA, and isobutyryl CoA. Insulin stimulates BCKAD kinase. BCKAD kinase is allosterically inhibited by the leucine substrate-α-ketoisocaproate, and inhibited by cortisol.

ammonium ion to the urea cycle and the remaining glutamate can then be transaminated to make aspartate, a crucial intermediate in the urea cycle. The last fate of glutamate in skeletal muscle is as a precursor in the formation of glutathione (Figure 12.7). Remember, glutathione is a key molecule in controlling reactive oxygen species (ROS) within the cell, by facilitating the conversion of H_2O_2 into H_2O.

Summary

As we exercise, we use three different energy systems: creatine phosphate, anaerobic glycolysis, and oxidative phosphorylation. The creatine phosphate system is exhausted in about the first 10–15 sec, leading to the increase of anaerobic glycolysis system, which dominates until about 2–3 minutes. Lastly, oxidative phosphorylation picks up and dominates from 2–3 minutes on. At rest and at low intensity exercise, fatty acid oxidation is the primary energy source. Remember, it takes about 20 min for fatty acids to become a major contributor. At about 50–65% VO_2 max, the cross-over point occurs, leading to an increase in glucose oxidation for intensities above this.

Exercise training leads to physiological changes all over the body including an increase in glycogen storage, mitochondrial number and oxidative enzymes, capillarization, muscle fiber types, and an increase in IMTGs and fat oxidation (moving the cross-over point to the right). Other changes include an increase in respiratory function, heart function, and systemic vascularization. Unfortunately, many of these changes can be ameliorated in just a week of detraining.

Calcium release during muscle contraction provides an alternative pathway for GLUT4 translocation, increasing glucose uptake, even in the absence of insulin. Glucose uptake is also stimulated after exercise without insulin and muscle is more insulin-sensitive than when it is in a resting state. Exercise is a crucial lifestyle change for diabetics.

BCAA catabolism provides amino acid carbon skeletons for use as energy, as well as producing glutamate. Glutamate can be used to clear nitrogen from muscle as it can be converted to glutamine, it can be used as the building blocked for the antioxidant glutathione, it can be used for protein synthesis, and it can be converted to alanine with pyruvate, providing an important gluconeogenic precursor to the liver. BCAA catabolism is regulated by the enzyme BCKAD, either by phosphorylation or allosteric modulators.

Points to Ponder

➢ Search the internet for papers discussing intramuscular triglycerides (IMTGs) and insulin resistance. What are some of the proposed pathways for IMTGs leading to insulin resistance?

➢ AMPK is proposed as a needed enzyme in the mitochondrial biogenesis pathway. What role do you think AMPK plays in this pathway?

➢ Which would be a better exercise protocol for weight loss? Running at 7.5 MPH for 30 min (high-intensity) or walking at 3.5 MPH for 60 min (low-intensity)? Find a "calories burned running" calculator and find out.

➢ Are calories burned during exercise the same for a 130 lb women as a 175 lb man, doing the same exercise for the same amount of time? Why do you think so?

➢ Would you ever consider creatine supplementation, why or why not? How about BCAA supplementation?

References

1. Hyde E, Omura, JD, Watson, KB, Fulton, JE, Carlson, SA. Knowledge of the Adult and Youth 2008 Physical Activity Guildlines for Americans. *Medicine and Science in Sports and Exercise.* 2018;50(5S):457.

2. Tucker JM, Welk GJ, Beyler NK. Physical activity in U.S.: adults compliance with the Physical Activity Guidelines for Americans. *Am J Prev Med.* 2011;40(4):454–461.

3. Berggren JR, Hulver MW, Dohm GL, Houmard JA. Weight loss and exercise: implications for muscle lipid metabolism and insulin action. *Med Sci Sports Exerc.* 2004;36(7):1191–1195.

4. Coen PM, Tanner CJ, Helbling NL, et al. Clinical trial demonstrates exercise following bariatric surgery improves insulin sensitivity. *J Clin Invest.* 2015;125(1):248–257.

5. Neufer PD, Bamman MM, Muoio DM, et al. Understanding the Cellular and Molecular Mechanisms of Physical Activity-Induced Health Benefits. *Cell Metab.* 2015;22(1):4–11.

6. Rueda-Clausen CF, Ogunleye AA, Sharma AM. Health Benefits of Long-Term Weight-Loss Maintenance. *Annu Rev Nutr.* 2015;35:475–516.

7. Jakicic JM. The effect of physical activity on body weight. *Obesity (Silver Spring).* 2009;17 Suppl 3:S34–38.

8. Wing RR, Phelan S. Long-term weight loss maintenance. *Am J Clin Nutr.* 2005;82(1 Suppl):222S-225S.

9. Volek JS, Kraemer WJ, Bush JA, et al. Creatine supplementation enhances muscular performance during high-intensity resistance exercise. *J Am Diet Assoc.* 1997;97(7):765–770.

10. Brooks GA, Mercier J. Balance of carbohydrate and lipid utilization during exercise: the "crossover" concept. *J Appl Physiol (1985).* 1994;76(6):2253–2261.

11. Ahmed K, Tunaru S, Tang C, et al. An autocrine lactate loop mediates insulin-dependent inhibition of lipolysis through GPR81. *Cell Metab.* 2010;11(4):311–319.

12. Putman CT, Jones NL, Hultman E, et al. Effects of short-term submaximal training in humans on muscle metabolism in exercise. *Am J Physiol.* 1998;275(1 Pt 1):E132–139.

13. Spencer MK, Yan Z, Katz A. Effect of low glycogen on carbohydrate and energy metabolism in human muscle during exercise. *Am J Physiol.* 1992;262(4 Pt 1):C975–979.

14. Hood DA, Uguccioni G, Vainshtein A, D'Souza D. Mechanisms of exercise-induced mitochondrial biogenesis in skeletal muscle: implications for health and disease. *Compr Physiol.* 2011;1(3):1119–1134.

15. Henriksson J. Effects of physical training on the metabolism of skeletal muscle. *Diabetes Care.* 1992;15(11):1701–1711.

16. Russell AP, Gastaldi G, Bobbioni-Harsch E, et al. Lipid peroxidation in skeletal muscle of obese as compared to endurance-trained humans: a case of good vs. bad lipids? *FEBS Lett.* 2003;551(1–3):104–106.

17. Heinonen I, Kalliokoski KK, Hannukainen JC, Duncker DJ, Nuutila P, Knuuti J. Organ-specific physiological responses to acute physical exercise and long-term training in humans. *Physiology (Bethesda).* 2014;29(6):421–436.

18. Whelton SP, Chin A, Xin X, He J. Effect of aerobic exercise on blood pressure: a meta-analysis of randomized, controlled trials. *Ann Intern Med.* 2002;136(7):493–503.

19. Terjung RL. Muscle adaptations to aerobic training. *Sports Science Exchange.* 54 (8):1.

20. Hearn GR. The effects of terminating and detraining on enzyme activities of heart and skeletal muscle of trained rats. *Int Z Angew Physiol.* 1965;21(3):190–194.

21. Neufer PD. The effect of detraining and reduced training on the physiological adaptations to aerobic exercise training. *Sports Med.* 1989;8(5):302–320.

22. Booth F. Effects of endurance exercise on cytochrome C turnover in skeletal muscle. *Ann N Y Acad Sci.* 1977;301:431–439.

23. Ryder JW, Chibalin AV, Zierath JR. Intracellular mechanisms underlying increases in glucose uptake in response to insulin or exercise in skeletal muscle. *Acta Physiol Scand.* 2001;171(3):249–257.

Carbohydrates

Forms

➤ Sugars: These are simple sugars such as glucose, dextrose, fructose.
➤ Sugar alcohols: These are molecules with sugar and alcohol components, such as sorbitol.
➤ Starches: Made up of long chains of linked glucose molecules, either amylose (non-branched) or amylopectin (branched).
➤ Dietary fiber: Includes both soluble and non-soluble fiber. Made up of many sugar molecules but they are branched with different bond orientations and not as easily digestible as starches.

Sources Carbohydrates are primarily found in plant sources, sugar, and in dairy products (lactose). This includes all the forms above, although many different sugar alcohols are produced commercially as reduced or no-calorie sweeteners. Simple sugars are also added to foods to change the taste or aid in texture or presentation. Good sources of starch and fibers include beans, peas, grains, and some vegetables such as carrots and potatoes.

Digestion Carbohydrate digestion occurs in the mouth and small intestine. In the mouth, salivary amylase begins breaking up starches. No digestion occurs in the stomach. In the small intestine, pancreatic amylase continues chopping up starches, and brush border enzymes finish the job. Maltase breaks down maltose, sucrase breaks down sucrose, lactase breaks down lactose, and isomaltase breaks down the branch points of amylopectin. Absorption occurs via specific monosaccharide carriers.

DRI Each gram of carbohydrate provides 4 Kcals of energy. The Recommended Daily Allowance (RDA) for total digestible carbohydrates is based on the role of carbohydrates as a primary source of energy for the brain. Adequate intake (AI) is indicated when an RDA is not available, and this includes all values for total fiber. The Acceptable Macronutrient Distribution Range (AMDR) is based on the role of digestible carbohydrates as a source of calories for maintaining body weight and preventing chronic disease[1]. ND-not determinable from available scientific research.

Total Digestible Carbohydrates[2]:

Life Stage	RDA (grams/day)	AMDR (% Kcals)
Infant (0–6 mo)	60 (AI)	ND
Infant (7–12 mo)	95 (AI)	ND
Children, Adults (1–70 years)	130	45–65
Pregnant Females	175	45–65
Lactating Females	210	45–65

Total Fiber[2]:

Life Stage	AI
Infant (0–12 mo)	ND
Children (1–3 years)	19
Children (4–8 years)	25
Males (9–13 years)	31
Males (14–50 years)	38
Males (50+ years)	30
Females (9–18 years)	26
Females (19–50 years)	25
Females (50+ years)	21
Pregnant Females	28
Lactating Females	29

Fats

Forms

➤ Saturated Fats: Usually solid at room temperature because they have no double bonds. That's where their name comes from because they are 'saturated' with hydrogen bonds. Examples include palmitic, stearic, lauric and myristic acid. These are not needed in the diet (there is no RDA/AI, but the American Heart Association recommends no more than 5–6% of Kcals should come from saturated fats).

➤ Unsaturated Fats: Are liquid at room temperature, except for some tropical sources such as palm oil and palm kernel oil, as these also contain hydrogenated oils, and saturated fats. These fat molecules have one or more double bonds. The more double bonds a fat has, the more susceptible it is to oxidation (and can become rancid at room temperature). These exist as cis- and trans- isomers, depending on the direction of the double bond.

  • Trans Fats: Not as common in natural products, these are produced commercially to stabilize foods. In nature, beef contains conjugated linoleic acids—a trans fat. CLA has both a cis-double bond, and a trans double bond, and may have some health benefits[3]. Elaidic acid is a trans fat, with the same chemical composition as oleic acid (a monounsaturated fat), but it is solid at room temperature.

  • Polyunsaturated Fats: These fats have more than one double bond and are liquid at room temperature. A common polyunsaturated fat is the omega-6 fatty acid, linoleic acid. Both omega 3s and omega 6s are essential polyunsaturated fats, that must come from the diet.

  • Monounsaturated Fats: These fats have one double bond. A common monounsaturated fat is oleic acid.

➤ Cholesterol: A waxy fat-like molecule produced by the liver which is not needed in the diet as the liver produces enough for the body's needs. There is no RDA/AI for cholesterol, however the American Heart Association, recommends less than 300 mg a day from dietary sources.

Sources Mono- and polyunsaturated fats are found in plants and seafood, while saturated and trans fats are found in animal products, processed foods such as meats, refrigerated dough, and desserts.

Digestion Fat digestion occurs in the mouth, stomach, and small intestine. In the mouth and stomach, lingual lipase and gastric lipase, respectively, begin digestion by removing one fatty acid from the triglyceride. In the small intestine, pancreatic lipase finishes digestion by producing free fatty acids and monoglycerides. Free fatty acids, monoglycerides, phospholipids, cholesterol, and fat-soluble vitamins are incorporated into a micelle for absorption.

DRI Each gram of fat provides 9 Kcal of energy. For adults, there is not a Recommended Daily Allowance (RDA) or an Adequate intake (AI) for fat because there is not enough data to confirm the level required for adequate health[1]. For infants, an AI has been developed. The Acceptable Macronutrient Distribution Range (AMDR) is based on the role fat as a source of calories for maintaining body weight [1]. For omega-6 and omega-3 fatty acids, AI have been established and are given. ND-not determinable from available scientific research.

Total Fat[2]:

Life Stage	AI (grams/day)	AMDR (% Kcals)
Infant (0–6 mo)	31	ND
Infant (7–12 mo)	30	ND
Children (1–3 years)	ND	30–40
Children (4–18)	ND	25–35
Adults (18+ years)	ND	20–35
Pregnant Females	ND	20–35
Lactating Females	ND	20–35

Omega-6 Polyunsaturated Fat (linoleic Acid)[2]:

Life Stage	AI (grams/day)	AMDR (% Kcals)
Infant (0–6 mo)	4.4	ND
Infant (7–12 mo)	4.6	ND
Children (1–3 years)	7	5–10
Children (4–8 years)	10	5–10
Males (9–13 years)	12	5–10
Males (14–18 years)	16	5–10
Males (19–50 years)	17	5–10
Males (50+ years)	14	5–10
Females (9–13 years)	10	5–10
Females (14–18 years)	11	5–10
Females (19–30 years)	12	5–10
Females (31+ years)	11	5–10
Pregnant Females	13	5–10
Lactating Females	13	5–10

Omega -3 Polyunsaturated Fat (alpha linolenic Acid)[2]:

Life Stage	AI (grams/day)	AMDR (% Kcal)
Infant (0–12 mo)	0.5	ND
Children (1–3 years)	0.7	0.6–1.2
Children (4–8 years)	0.9	0.6–1.2
Males (9–13 years)	1.2	0.6–1.2
Males (14+ years)	1.6	0.6–1.2
Females (9–13 years)	1.0	0.6–1.2
Females (14+ years)	1.1	0.6–1.2
Pregnant Females	1.4	0.6–1.2
Lactating Females	1.3	0.6–1.2

Proteins

Forms From the common phrase, "one gene = one protein" there should be at least 20,000 proteins, but we know there are many, many more than this, as one gene can make several different protein isoforms, and in some cases, even completely different proteins. One recent paper claims that one average gene could make up to 100 different proteins if alternative splicing, alternative start and stop sites, and gene/mRNA editing all occur in that single gene[4]. No one wants to state the exact number of proteins that any organism can make, so we won't either. Proteins are made from a chain of amino acids, which can be divided into two main groups:

➤ Essential Amino Acids: These are amino acids that are essential in the diet—either the body cannot make them in sufficient quantities or does not make them at all. Nine amino acids are essential. They are histidine, isoleucine, leucine, lysine, methionine, phenylalanine, threonine, tryptophan, and valine.

➤ Non-essential Amino Acids: These amino acids do not have to be part of a normal diet, as the body can make them from other building blocks, including recycled proteins. Eleven amino acids are considered non-essential. They are alanine, asparagine, aspartate, cysteine, glutamate, glutamine, glycine, proline, serine, tyrosine, and arginine.

Sources Proteins are found in all types of foods, including beans, peas, and animal products. Sources include dairy, nuts, seeds, grains, soy, and some vegetables (although these generally contain less protein).

Digestion Protein digestion occurs in the stomach and small intestine. In the stomach the enzyme pepsin chops up proteins into oligopeptides. In the small intestine, trypsin, chymotrypsin, carboxy-peptidases, and elastin break the oligopeptides into single amino acids, di- and tripeptides. Brush border enzymes finish the job. Dipeptidase, tripeptidase, and aminopeptidases produce single amino acids and dipeptides, which are absorbed via specific amino acid carriers and dipeptide carriers.

DRI Each gram of protein provides 4 Kcal of energy. The Recommended Daily Allowance (RDA) for total protein is 0.8 g per Kg body weight. The RDA in the following table is based on the role of proteins in whole body nitrogen balance studies (catabolism/anabolism of proteins). The Acceptable Macronutrient Distribution Range (AMDR) is based on the role of proteins as a source of Kcals for maintaining body weight[1]. ND-not determinable from available scientific research.

Total Protein[2]

Life Stage	RDA (grams/day)	AMDR (% Kcals)
Infant (0–6 mo)	9.1 (AI)	ND
Infant (7–12 mo)	11.0	ND
Children (1–3 years)	13	5–20
Children (4–8 years)	19	10–30
Males (9–13 years)	34	10–30
Males (14–18 years)	52	10–30
Males (19+ years)	56	10–35
Females (9–13)	34	10–30
Females (14+)	46	10–35
Pregnant and Lactating Females	71	10–35

RDA for Essential Amino Acids

Amino Acid	mg/kg Body Weight (US values)	mg/kg Body Weight (WHO values)
Histidine	14	10
Isoleucine	19	20
Leucine	42	39
Lysine	38	30
Methionine (+cysteine)	19	15
Phenylalanine (+tyrosine)	33	25
Threonine	20	15
Tryptophan	5	4
Valine	24	26

References

1. Medicine Io. Dietary Reference Intakes: The Essential Guide to Nutrient Requirements. Washington DC: The National Academies Press; 2006.

2. Institute of Medicine (U.S.). Panel on Macronutrients., Institute of Medicine (U.S.). Standing Committee on the Scientific Evaluation of Dietary Reference Intakes. *Dietary reference intakes for energy, carbohydrate, fiber, fat, fatty acids, cholesterol, protein, and amino acids.* Washington, D.C.: National Academies Press; 2005.

3. Dilzer A, Park Y. Implication of conjugated linoleic acid (CLA) in human health. *Crit Rev Food Sci Nutr.* 2012;52(6):488–513.

4. Ponomarenko EA, Poverennaya EV, Ilgisonis EV, et al. The Size of the Human Proteome: The Width and Depth. *Int J Anal Chem.* 2016;2016:7436849.